MW01169707

Choose Health

Dr. L. Scott Monk

ISBN 0-7414-1863-0

Published by:

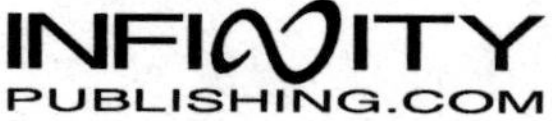

519 West Lancaster Avenue
Haverford, PA 19041-1413
Info@buybooksontheweb.com
www.buybooksontheweb.com
Toll-free (877) BUY BOOK
Local Phone (610) 520-2500
Fax (610) 519-0261

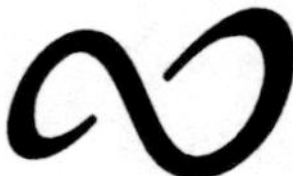

Printed in the United States of America

Printed on Recycled Paper

Published January 2004

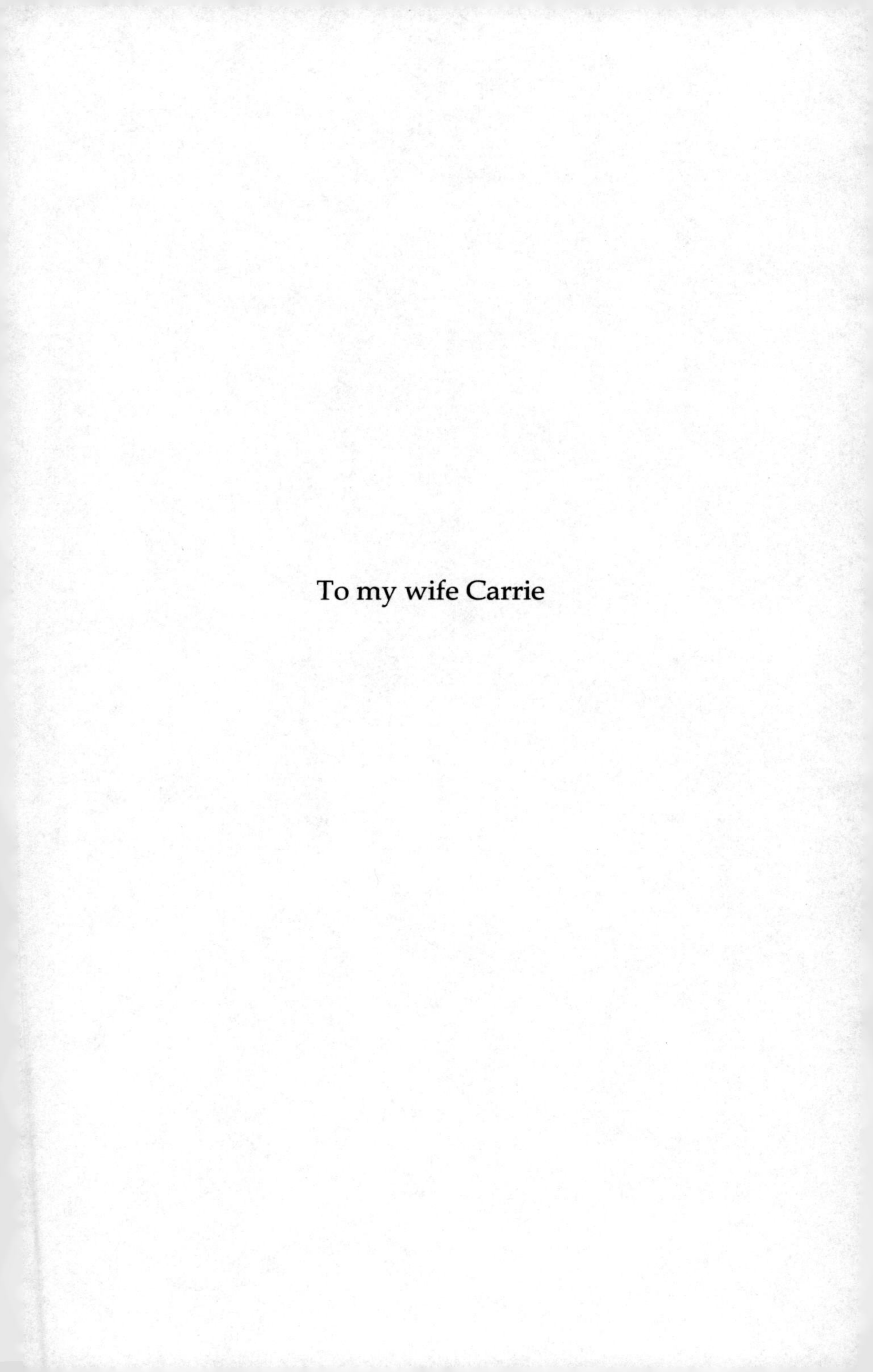

To my wife Carrie

Special thanks to:

Melissa Martin
&
Kristin Schrader

FOREWORD .... *A*

INTRODUCTION *1*

SECTION I: IN THE OFFICE* *0

MY PHILOSOPHY *1*

HEALTH QUESTIONNAIRE *17*

APPLIED KINESIOLOGY *22*

STRUCTURAL THERAPIES *31*

Spinal Adjustments 32

Vector Point Cranial Therapy 34

Cranial Sacral Therapy 36

Exercise Programs 38

Orthopedic Supports 40

NUTRITIONAL THERAPIES *42*

Diet 43

Supplementation 45

Detoxification 47

EMOTIONAL THERAPIES *50*

ENERGETIC THERAPIES *53*

LABORATORY EXAMINATIONS *57*

SECTION II: COMMON CHRONIC CONDITIONS* *64

CHRONIC ILLNESS PROTOCOL *65*

ALLERGIES *73*

STRESS *77*

WOMEN'S HEALTH *84*

Hormone Replacement Therapy (Hrt) 84

Menstrual Irregularities 93

Pre Menstrual Syndrome (Pms) 93

Menopause 95

Depression 96

Osteoporosis 99

Balancing Estrogen 101

HYPOGLYCEMIA *103*

CHOLESTEROL *106*

CANDIDA *113*

PAIN *117*

LOW BACK PAIN *120*

WEIGHT LOSS *126*

SECTION III: AT HOME 138

DIET & FOODS 139

DETOXIFICATION 155

Supplements 158
Exercise 159
Colon Cleansing 160
Do-It-Yourself Formulas For The Colon 162
Liver Cleansing 164
Kidney Cleansing 166
Skin Cleansing 166
Fasting 167

PREPARING FOODS 169

Grains, Nuts & Seeds 169
Sprouting Grains & Seeds 169
Soaking Grains & Nuts 170
Grain Mills 170

MILK 172

HEALTH CABINET 173

CARING FOR CHILDREN 185

Before Birth 186
Newborns 189
Breast Milk Quality 190
Dietary Guidelines For Children 193
Common Problems With Kids 201
Colic 201
Ear Infections 202
Vaccinations 203

Treating Sick Kids 209

EXERCISE 214

Fitness Vs. Health 214
The Anaerobic System 215
The Aerobic System 216
Target Heart Rate 218
The Emotional Component 220
Warm Up, Cool Down And Stretching 221
Maximum Aerobic Function Test (Maf) 222

SELF TREATMENT 224

Step I - Collect A Body Sample 227
Step II – Sample Placement 227
Step III – The Emotional Component 227
Step IV – The Neurolymphatic Reflexes 227
Step VI – Repeat Steps Iv & V 228

SECTION IV: RESOURCES ... **231**

YEAST DIET ... *232*

RECIPES ... *235*

Eggs ... 237
Pork & Turkey ... 240
Salads ... 242
Chicken ... 245
Soups ... 248
Beef ... 251
Other ... 253

TRACKING SHEETS ... *255*

Toxicity Self Test ... 257
Mediclear ... 259
Target Heart Rate ... 260
Maximum Aerobic Function Test ... 261
Progress Tracking Sheet ... 262

TESTIMONIALS ... *263*

ADDITIONAL SOURCES ... *267*

Websites ... 268
Books ... 271

BIBLIOGRAPHY ... *276*

INDEX ... *279*

FOREWORD

Melissa Martin

When Dr. Monk asked me to write the foreword for his second book, I was incredibly honored. Once I left his office and was driving home, I became very excited at the prospect of perhaps, in some small way, influencing the lives and health of others for the better. As I sat down to begin composing my thoughts, I was overwhelmed. I thought to myself, "You have never written a foreword. What were you thinking? You are neither a writer nor a practitioner of complementary medicine. What do you have to add to this book?" In the midst of my slowly mounting panic, I realized why Dr. Monk had asked me to do this. I am healed. I am living proof that the information presented in this book, if put to practice in your life, is powerful for the recovery of health and vitality. Let me share with you my story.

I was perhaps 12 or 13 years old when I developed a chronic strep infection in my throat. Over the next 2-3 years I was repeatedly placed on antibiotics to combat the infection. In just under 3 years I went through more than 15 rounds of antibiotics. When pharmaceutical drug treatment failed to effectively deal with the strep infection, the next step was to remove my tonsils. However, even after my tonsillectomy my health did not improve. I did not get strep throat as frequently as I used to, although I still came down with a strep infection periodically. Instead, I contracted other kinds of infections, from the common cold (several times a year) to bronchitis to vaginal yeast infections. Additionally, many of my symptoms continued to worsen. These included extreme fatigue, joint and muscle pain, digestive issues, headaches, menstrual cramps, severe mood swings, depression, difficulty concentrating, memory problems and a host of others.

Over the next 12 or so years I saw a virtual parade of doctors, specialists and even a psychologist for depression and suicidal thoughts. I was diagnosed with fibromyalgia, chronic fatigue syndrome and soft-tissue rheumatism. When I was 22 years old, one specialist told me that it was her professional opinion that I was at high risk of developing Lupus in a few years time. (She had no practical advice as to how I could avoid that particular fatal disease.) I was treated with drugs. I was told that there was nothing at all wrong with me and that the problems were all in my head. I was treated with more drugs. I was even physically manipulated by one doctor to produce symptoms that indicated the diagnosis that he wanted to make. In short, I had experiences with conventional medicine and traditional doctors that, sadly, I believe are far, far too common today.

Over the years I rode a vicious wave of sickness. I became disillusioned with doctors and fed up with drugs. It was the grace of God that led me to Dr. Monk and that enjoined me to hope, just one more time, that this doctor, at last, would be one who could help me. When I came to Dr. Monk's office I had been sick for over a dozen years and I had suffered under the care of almost as many physicians. My first visit to his office was a new experience for me in a number of ways. I had never before seen a doctor of complementary medicine. I knew relatively little about alternative medicine, though I would do much research in the following months. Also, I had never truly been *listened* to. Previous doctors would hear my list of complaints and jot down notes, but they universally tuned out when I began to share what I actually thought about my condition, especially if I indicated that I had done any kind of research on my own. One of the foremost things that I respect and appreciate about Dr. Monk is that he communicates with his patients. He asked intelligent questions about my symptoms and what I thought about my condition. He respectfully listened to my thoughts and encouraged further research on my part. If I was in error with something that I said, he explained why. That was an enormous change for me: a doctor not only willing but proactive in explaining why I was the way that I was, how the body functions and how his treatments would help my body overcome sickness. By far, the most profound new experience that I had during my first visit with Dr. Monk, something that no one else had ever done and a moment that I will never forget, was when he looked directly into my eyes and said "...you will get better."

After one month under Dr. Monk's care I was healthier than I could ever remember feeling in my life. I had lived under the weight and shadow of illness for so long that I had forgotten what it felt like to be well. I recall Dr. Monk asking me after my first several visits to gauge my progress: was I at about 60%, 75%? How much had I improved under the protocol that he had designed? I thought for a long minute before I replied, "I don't know." I did not know what 'healthy' felt like. I had no reference point in my memory to measure my progress against. Additionally, I had been ill for so long that I also forgot what 'sick' felt like. It sounds like a paradox, but I believe it to be a truth that is clearly visible in our society if you know what to look for. When one lives with illness or dysfunction day after day for months and years, one's perception of sickness changes. It is precisely because we first lose touch with our reference point of true health that we begin to perceive sickness in a different, skewed way. For much of the 12 years that I was sick I might have said that I was at perhaps 80% of optimal health. Looking back now, with my new understanding of health, I know without a doubt that I was never over 50% in all of those years, excepting a brief period of a few months when I was at perhaps 70%.

In the end it did not matter. When I was really and truly well, I knew it. I was a different person in every way: physically, spiritually, mentally and emotionally. I do not know if it is like that for everyone, but that was how I knew that I was well. Thus began my journey not only into restored health but also into a renewed life. I began to research what complementary healthcare was all about. What I found astounded me. Alternative treatments are misunderstood and much maligned by many in the traditional medical field. Nonetheless, if you take the time to research these things honestly, thoroughly, and with an open mind you will find as I did, that alternative medicine is highly effective. I came to realize, both from my own experience and from the information I had researched, that this type of medicine is truly the optimal form of healthcare because it treats and cares for people, not diseases, and because it focuses on prevention. It is an individualized, whole-person approach. After all, you are not exactly like anyone else on Earth, nor are you merely a compilation of symptoms. You are unique: body, mind and spirit. Complementary medicine sees you and treats you as such.

I will warn you now that *Choose Health* will not give you a 'quick fix' or easy remedy for your health issues. You must be responsible for your own health. This does not mean that you yourself need to be able to treat everything that goes wrong. That is absurd. It does mean that you need to educate yourself about how your body works, how to maintain your health and how to deal with sickness. It also requires that you be informed when choosing doctors or alternative healthcare practitioners. Ask them questions, and not just "Yes" or "No" questions. Ask them hard questions. Get to know them before you place your life and health in their hands. Finally, you need to be willing to work at it. Contrary to what many pharmaceutical commercials would have you believe, no "wonder drug" will restore your health and make everything better. God willing, you will restore your health, in partnership with the healthcare practitioner(s) that you have chosen.

Choose Health is a powerful resource that will equip you with the information that you need to begin making a positive difference for your own health. Dr. Monk describes many of the chronic conditions that he sees in his office every week as well as some of the causes of these conditions. He explains the highly effective treatments that he uses as a Chiropractor and Applied Kinesiologist to help people overcome illness. He includes detailed information on nutrition and exercise and how these aspects of health need to be incorporated into individual protocols. The Self-Help and At Home sections explain what you can specifically do for yourself to improve your health. In essence, *Choose Health* is both an educational tool and practical tool.

Choose Health will also give you insight into Dr. Monk's philosophy of health and his view on many healthcare issues. His style is warm and personable. His approach is straightforward. Without fail, Dr. Monk deals with me honestly, compassionately and expertly. You will find him to be the same within the pages of his book. It is my fervent hope that you take this information and apply it to your life. You do not have to be sick, in pain or on drugs for the rest of your days. There is a better way.

INTRODUCTION

Be transformed by the renewing of your mind.
Romans 12

There is a healthcare crisis in this country. While insurance coverage, prescription drug benefits, and rising healthcare costs are genuine concerns, the healthcare crisis I refer to is a lack of fundamental knowledge about one's health. In general, people in this country know very little about their bodies; how they function, how they prevent sickness and how they recover from illness. As a result, people are utterly dependent upon a health care system that has little to do with preventing illness or maintaining health, but is entirely driven by combating disease. Frankly, there is just no money to be made in disease prevention.

The topic of health is further complicated by many factors. The human body is complex to say the least, making an exhaustive study impractical. Diseases are difficult to understand and contain. Remedies and techniques vary from place to place and from doctor to doctor. The health care industry is a competitive business with each faction vying for its share of the illness market, which often leads to misinformation and exaggeration. Countless books have been written on hundreds of health-related subjects, both clarifying and confusing issues, creating a state of information paralysis. Just which "expert" does one believe? Despite many decent attempts at explaining and simplifying these issues, confusion abounds.

Those good souls in the medical field who do teach and promote some form of prevention, too often come from a singular perspective and are therefore not familiar with the effects of their approach on the body as a whole. For example, weight loss can be beneficial but empty calories from over processed foods will irritate stressed-out organs and tissues. Likewise, exercise to the point of exhaustion may make you physically fit (vs. *healthy*), but it may also create panic attacks, night sweats and other symptoms resulting from hormonal imbalances.

I have spent the last ten years or so as a patient, student and now doctor of complimentary medicine. As such, I have been exposed to and use techniques that address the entire body, not just a single part. With every treatment plan, I do my best to make sure that it is beneficial for the patient as a whole. Goals are placed within the context of generating health.

So, you want to climb a mountain? Great, let's make sure that your nutritional reserves are built up before you begin hiking 3 hours a day and then quit because of aching joints that won't heal. You want to lose 30 pounds? Great, let's make sure you are detoxified from years of a poor diet before we reduce calories and begin an exercise program that can place too much stress on your liver. However, skilled treatment plans and good intentions are not enough.

I have come to realize that there are four reasons why people are not healthy. 1. They live in ignorance, not knowing the truth; 2. They live in denial, not accepting the truth; 3. They live in deception – believing something other than the truth; 4. They live as they decide to, creating their own truth. Let me illustrate.

I will never forget an experience I had while giving a lecture. The meeting was held at a fitness center in a neighboring town. 18 or so people were crowded into a small room to hear my talk, *The Metabolic Stumbling Blocks to Losing Weight*.

About half way through I was interrupted by a gentleman sitting off to the side. Up to that point I noticed that he didn't often make eye-contact, instead he seemed preoccupied with the printed material and was meticulously going through it. This seemed like a positive sign at the time – the behavior of someone genuinely interested in learning something new. He asked what a certain sentence was supposed to say on a particular slide which read,

"Avoid highly processed luncheon meats and sausage containing and other additives."

It was evident that I had made a typographical error and omitted a word or two. I thanked him for finding the error and turned to continue my presentation. He then spoke up again, "I found a few other mistakes as well, punctuation mostly." The situation was becoming clear to me as I have encountered attitudes like this before. I then made some sort of joke to keep the mood light.

After my presentation this gentleman came over to talk. Before saying a word he pointed to his handout and showed me a circled word, "florescent". To his dismay, I had misspelled the word "fluorescent". I tried to keep a pleasant mood and made a joke about upgrading the "spell check" on my computer. He didn't laugh. Finally, in order to be more direct, I not-so-jokingly said, "I hope you found more in this talk than just grammatical errors." This seemed to have some effect as he then began to share "his story." Everyone has a story.

He described how he was raised, "In my family you had to finish what was on your plate. So now I clean my plate at restaurants, which is food enough for two days." Evidently, he was trying to blame his parents, restaurants or both for his weight problem. This man then said, "You were talking about different foods, good ones and bad ones. Well if it tastes good that means it is 'good', and if it tastes bad, that means it is 'bad". I responded, "You don't believe that. You have a brain, the ability to learn and the ability to choose. It doesn't matter how you were raised. When you decide that you are going to make beneficial changes you will. Until then you can hide behind excuses if you choose, but if you want to know why you have a weight problem look in the mirror."

This book is a concentrated course in health, meant to enlighten, educate and empower those who would choose to learn.

SECTIONS I & II, are what I, as a complimentary (alternative) doctor, do to heal the sick and prevent illness. You will learn about subtle and effective techniques that produce significant, positive health results. You will also be exposed to my personal philosophy of health - a common sense approach. SECTION III is the self-help portion. It is designed to help current patients and people who would otherwise not be able to come into the office for a visit. Many will find this section very challenging. However, if put to proper use this material will change the way you think, and perhaps change the way you live your life as well. Enjoy!

IN THE OFFICE

SECTION I

MY PHILOSOPHY

This chapter is essential to your future if you are at all interested in achieving and maintaining health. In an easy to understand way, I will explain how the body works, why it gets sick, and how it recovers from illness. My ideas are in conflict with mainstream or traditional medical philosophy. Therefore it is necessary to discuss these differences first. Seeing the contrasts for yourself will help you make informed decisions about your health. The philosophy I describe here is based on answering the common question, "Why am I sick?" Believe it or not, many traditionally trained doctors cannot answer this most basic of questions. The same is true for most people. It is as if fate alone, and not lifestyle choices were the sole reason for illness. This type of thinking is a direct result of the disease model of healthcare ascribed to by most medical doctors.

In the disease model all resources are devoted to the detection and elimination of a definable disease. This philosophy is greatly flawed and results in limited treatment options (drugs or surgery) and gullible patients. It also produces arrogant doctors who see the disease model as the only valid approach. This model is also powerless to help people with significant symptoms, but no sign of recognizable disease, what I call *functional illness*. If a disease cannot be found then, "It must be in your head." Many of my patients have been told this repeatedly only to see their health restored again when a natural, whole person approach was undertaken.

One of the tragic effects of the disease model is the control of patients and their choices. When a diagnosis is assigned by traditional doctors, most patients will take whatever medications they are prescribed without so much as a pause to consider what and why, consoling themselves with thoughts like, "Well he's the doctor, he knows best." It is true, the doctor should know what he or she is doing and should also know more about health and sickness than you, but that does not let you off the hook. In fact, it leaves you in an extremely vulnerable position.

On a brighter note, I am greatly encouraged by the number of new patients that come in to my office who do know a good deal about their symptoms or conditions and how they came to be. I believe this is the result of three things, the access to information via the internet, the growth of complimentary medicine and the emergence of wise non-traditional medical doctors. This book is an attempt to further this positive trend.

The Philosophy

There are many aspects to understanding the health of the human body. I begin by contrasting the two dominant views, Traditional vs. Alternative, and then describe certain details in a common sense manner. Below I have listed the topics in order.

- Different Approaches
- The Strength of Traditional Medicine
- The Weaknesses of Traditional Medicine
- The Growth of Alternative Medicine
- My Health Philosophy
- Prevention Is the Key
- The Human Body Is Complex
- The Human Body Is Sensitive
- The Human Body Heals Itself
- The Human Body's Health Is Conditional
- The Human Body Constantly Adapts To Stress
- The Human Body's Incredible Resistance
- The Human Body Is Interconnected
- The Human Body Prioritizes Stress

Different Approaches

All health care providers can be placed into either one of two groups. The first group, Traditional physicians consists of medical doctors and osteopaths. The second group, complimentary or alternative health practitioners is made up of chiropractors, acupuncturists, massage therapists, herbalists, homeopaths, naturopaths and more. These two groups do not think alike. As I mentioned above, there are exceptions; MD's who use herbs, refer patients to chiropractors, employ an acupuncturist and so on, but these are still few.

Each type of health care has its place. I am not against traditional medicine. I believe in the use of pharmaceutical drugs and in the use of surgery when warranted. However, I am greatly opposed to the misuse of drugs and surgery, which has resulted from the traditional medicine belief that theirs is the best and only remedy. The key is, knowing when to use which kind of medicine. It is not good doctoring to have surgery to remove a gall bladder when a simple supplement taken for three weeks and a change in diet would have done the trick. In the same way, getting an adjustment to correct a ruptured appendix is just as foolish and possibly deadly. As a new student of health, it is important to understand the differences between the two schools of thought.

Alternative Health Care Beliefs	**Traditional (Medical) Health Care Beliefs**
Diseases are natural, a symptom that the body is not functioning well.	Diseases are unnatural and should be vigorously fought against.
The body is a whole. When any part suffers it is a symptom that the body is not functioning properly.	The body is a combination of parts. When a part is damaged it can be repaired, removed or replaced.
Diet is a key to correcting current and preventing future illness.	Diet receives very little consideration in most illnesses.
Nutritional supplements or herbs are extremely important for overall health.	Supplements are not important. Eating a "balanced" diet (if diet is discussed) is what's important.

Sickness or diseases may be treated with any therapy (adjustments, herbs, acupuncture needles, sensory stimulation etc.) directed at restoring overall chemical, structural, emotional or energetic balance.	Surgery and drugs are the primary means of treatments.

Figure I

From these two lists, you can see why medical doctors do not often agree with the ideas and approaches of chiropractors, acupuncturists and other alternative physicians. This is only the beginning of the confusion.

If you were to ask a medical doctor, a chiropractor, an acupuncturist, and a homeopath the same question, "What causes the common cold?" you would undoubtedly get four different answers. Not only that, but you will probably get four different treatments as well.

The Strength of Traditional Medicine

I believe traditional medicine has gained such a strong foothold for a number of reasons. First of all, medicine can and has done a great deal of good. Many diseases have been eliminated or held at bay thanks to the efforts of modern medicine. These facts are not overlooked. Beyond that, medicine is easy for the patient. The idea of taking a pill to cure your symptoms or lying asleep on a table and then waking up better is very appealing. There is little or no effort involved – a pleasant thought for many in our society. Also, medicine is exciting, even glamorous. Just think, any day now there may be a new medical breakthrough or cure for one of the world's most heinous diseases. Imagine of all the scientists in all the major universities around the world peering through their microscopes, testing new compounds, and making new discoveries. No wonder medical doctors are so revered. Consider all of the Hollywood celebrities raising money to find a cure for this or that disease. Participation in the funding of scientific research allows the public to be part of the movement to find a cure. Next, insurance pays for traditional medicine. Most people in our society have some form of insurance coverage through work, a spouse, Medicare or Medicaid. I know many people who will not even try alternative medicine because their insurance will not cover it. They can buy a new car every two years, send their kids to private school, and have season tickets to see the football team, but to pay out-of-pocket for alternative medicine is unthinkable. Many will not even consider alternatives because of a final reason. Traditional medicine has the mind of the public.

Most people still think about their primary care physician first. I don't know how many times I have had to convince a patient that I can help a disc bulge in their lower back or neck, even though spinal adjustments have been repeatedly shown to be the best form of treatment. They sheepishly ask, "Do you think you can help me with my problem?" "It is one of the things I do everyday." I reply. "Oh, really, I have been to my doctor and the physical therapist for the last six weeks and haven't gotten any better." If it weren't for motivation through desperation I suppose some people would just lie in bed and suffer if their MD couldn't help. The captured mind is a huge obstacle to overcome in any field.

The Weaknesses of Traditional Medicine

Economics, politics and other powerful forces are at work preventing certain ideas from becoming known while glorifying others. This is true for almost any established field of business. Yes, medicine is a business. To prove this point you only need watch any national news program and count the number of pharmaceutical advertisements and news stories having to do with some new medical breakthrough. If all these medical breakthroughs were viable we would have been freed from disease decades ago.

Today's hospitals, with all of their wonderful and life-saving advancements are also a good example of the weaknesses of traditional medicine. According to the Journal of the American Medical Association (JAMA), July 26th, 2000 (Vol. 284, No. 4) issue, in the United States there are approximately:

- 12,000 deaths annually from unnecessary surgery.
- 7,000 deaths annually from medication errors.
- 20,000 deaths annually from other errors in hospitals.

- 80,000 deaths annually from nosocomial infections (infections acquired in a hospital).
- 106,000 deaths annually from non-error, adverse effects of medications.

"These total to 225,000 deaths per year from iatrogenic causes [resulting from the doctor]." These estimates are for deaths only and do not include adverse effects associated with disability or discomfort.

225,000 deaths constitutes the third leading cause of death in the United States, after deaths from heart disease and cancer. Even when death was not an issue, the article went on to estimate that between 4 and 18 percent of hospital patients experienced adverse effects resulting in:

- 116 million extra patient visits.
- 77 million extra prescriptions.
- 17 million emergency department visits.
- 8 million hospitalizations.
- 3 million long-term admissions.
- And $77 billion in extra costs.

You might be thinking that this is the price we have to pay in our industrialized society, but that is not necessarily the case. Japan ranks second only to the United States in the number of advanced diagnostic equipment, like MRI and CT. However, Japan ranks highest on health, whereas the United States ranks among the lowest. The author explains this by noting that the results of the diagnostic imaging often result in the American patient being hospitalized. Conversely, in Japan the common practice is to have the family members provide the amenities of hospital care.

As I mentioned earlier, the healthcare system in United States is not a health care system at all. Instead it is a disease care system. I am not sure of all the reasons why home care is statistically better than hospital care. Is it the personal attention, the kindness of family members, the food, the emotional comfort or some combination? What is clear is that to avoid becoming a statistic like those mentioned above, the best thing to do is to avoid the hospital by avoiding disease through prevention.

The Growth of Alternative Medicine

Patients who have chosen alternative medicine either instinctively noticed the problems with traditional medicine or have experienced them first hand. Alternative health care has continued to grow steadily for the last thirty years in spite of all of the strengths of traditional medicine. Patients have spoken with their wallets, choosing to pay around $30 billion annually for alternative care, most of which is not covered by their insurance carriers. This fact has not gone undetected.

I saw a special "Health Report" on the news describing an electronic devise worn on the wrist. Its purpose was to decrease the nausea experienced by cancer patients. The reporter went into great detail explaining how it works, touting the wonderful potential benefits. Little did she know that the devise was stimulating a well-known point on an acupuncture meridian. Of course, no acupuncture terminology was used and no credit was given. To control nausea, acupuncture patients have used similar non-electronic wristbands for years at a cost of around $5.00. This devise sold for $150.00. So we see that the resistance to embrace non-traditional forms of medicine is still great. Recognition and acceptance are not in the minds of traditional doctors, rather acquisition and absorption.

As a result of the demand by satisfied patients, traditional medicine has reluctantly "accepted" some forms of alternative treatment for specific conditions: acupuncture for pain, chiropractic for lower back problems and massage therapy for stress. Prior to this the only answer given for treatments that worked but were not pharmaceutically based was the placebo effect. In other words, the patient so greatly believed that they would get better; they did, through a mysterious process in their own minds. Though the placebo effect is a real phenomenon, it was inadequate as the sole explanation for all of the benefits achieved through alternative health care. Interestingly, since alternative health care providers are often the last of many doctors to be visited for the same condition, doesn't it seem strange that the placebo effect took so long to happen? Or, put another way, why didn't the placebo effect occur when the medical treatments were given?

My Health Philosophy

As one might guess from the information above, the answer to the question, "What is health?" depends upon whom you ask. The philosophies of health are vast and intimately related to many factors including: cultural and religious beliefs, education, and economics. In fact, many philosophies running throughout health care are in direct conflict with one another. This means they cannot all be true at the same time. The most accurate health philosophy must address all possibilities that may potentially influence one's health.

In the paragraphs below, I have arrived at what I believe is an acceptable and accurate philosophy of health given what we know today. It takes bits and pieces from several different ideas and is applicable for any patient under any circumstance. However, because of our designed complexity, the ideas below are in no way exhaustive...but they are a good start.

Prevention is the Key

The war-on-cancer has been in effect for decades and has done very little to increase the effectiveness of cancer treatments or decrease the rates of cancer in general. In fact, cancer rates are much worse. The same is true for heart disease and almost any other top-ten killer. In my opinion the disease model, the approach used in the war-on-cancer, is flawed from the start because it completely neglects the body's own disease fighting ability; relegating all of the responsibility for overcoming disease to a surgeon or a pill.

Preventing illness is clearly the best option for many reasons. It allows for an extended quality of life; it enhances the functional life of all people; it places responsibility on the patient – accepting responsibility for ourselves and our actions is beneficial not only for health reasons but also for society in general. Finally, it is the least expensive – with our current health care crisis, this should be appealing.

To illustrate the difference between the prevention model and the disease model I have chosen the topic of high blood pressure.

Millions of Americans have this condition and are placed on blood pressure lowering medication everyday. Is this the right approach? High blood pressure has many causes including:

- Dehydration
- Toxicity
- Arteriosclerosis
- Nervousness
- Autonomic nervous system imbalance
- Food allergies
- Nutritional imbalances
- Kidney stress and more.

I have lowered the blood pressure of patients by 10 to 20 points in the office simply by doing a few corrective procedures. The right supplements can have a profound effect as well – indicating a deficiency. Walking 20-30 minutes each day and simply drinking more water are both a tremendous help. My question is this: If any or all of these other options lower blood pressure, why is it that medical doctors only prescribe medication?

Here is another thought: Is high blood pressure always bad? If you are toxic, the body simply increases blood pressure so that you will remove the toxins faster. If you are dehydrated you need to move the thickened blood through the vessels faster so that oxygen and other nutrients are available. In these and other cases, could not high blood pressure simply be a sign indicating some sort of dysfunction? The answer is "yes". Therefore, if there were good reasons for the presence of high blood pressure, wouldn't it be detrimental to lower it?

The Human Body Is Complex

The human body is made up first of all with atoms (perhaps even something smaller or non-visible), then molecules, then cells, then tissues, then organs, then systems, and finally, you. Each part is built from smaller parts but even the smallest part has incredible complexity. It is interesting to note that many scientists when discussing a cell describe it as, "the basic structure of a living organism." And yet there is not one "basic" thing about it. A single human cell is more complex than all of New York City. And there are more than 100 trillion cells in your body! The diversity and specificity of a cell's individual components is staggering. A single cell must be able to exist as an individual structure and as part of a complex. It must produce energy, exchange chemicals, maintain homeostasis, resist attack from foreign invaders (viruses & bacteria), and reproduce. Each of these aspects is fully incomprehensible on its own. "Basic?" Definitely not.

The Human Body is Sensitive

Another example of the body's complexity is the central nervous system. It is composed of an estimated 100 billion neurons. It receives literally millions of bits of information from different sensory organs and then integrates all of these to determine the response made by the body. Most activities of the nervous system are initiated by sensory experience emanating from sensory receptors, whether visual receptors (sight), auditory receptors (sound), olfactory receptors (smell), tactile receptors (touch) or others. The student of physiology learns that this sensory experience can cause an immediate reaction, or its memory can be stored in the brain for minutes, weeks or even years. Depending upon the circumstances, a seemingly minor sensory stimulus can have a lasting physical or psychological impact.

The Human Body Heals Itself

In chiropractic school I was taught that the body has an innate intelligence. That is to say, each person has a built-in healing mechanism. Most health care providers would agree with this idea. Alternative health care providers go a bit further and believe that because of these built-in mechanisms, it is the human body that is best able to correct itself given the right sort of push. I agree with this. I sum it up to my patients by suggesting that God knew what he was doing when he put us together.

The Human Body's Health is Conditional

Despite these built in mechanisms to keep us going, we all eventually fall apart. The health of our bodies is conditional. There are choices to be made. In the long and sometimes short run, bad choices mean less vitality, while good choices mean more vitality. Not all decisions however, are equal for each person. As an example, the choice to eat dairy products may go well with you but not go well with me. We each have different strengths and weaknesses.

The Human Body Constantly Adapts to Stress

Have you ever wondered why one person gets asthma, and another gets migraines? Why is one family member healthy while the other is a walking medicine cabinet? As we learned earlier in this chapter, countless numbers of stimuli such as sounds, smells, tastes, stimulants, sensations etc., are bombarding our nervous system moment by moment. Too much of any stimuli at any given time can become a stress. The energy required to recognize, process and in some cases eliminate these stimuli is enormous. For these reasons, adaptation may be defined as: *the process of managing stress so that the body may exist in its most efficient state*. In other words, your body does the best it can with what it has, given the circumstances.

Mention the word stress and most people think of too many hours at work, a pregnant mom, trouble in relationships or other emotionally taxing circumstances. However, stress can be much more than that. In fact stress can result from almost anything. Put simply, stress is either too much of a bad thing (toxicity) or not enough of a good thing (deficiency). The chart below breaks it down even further.

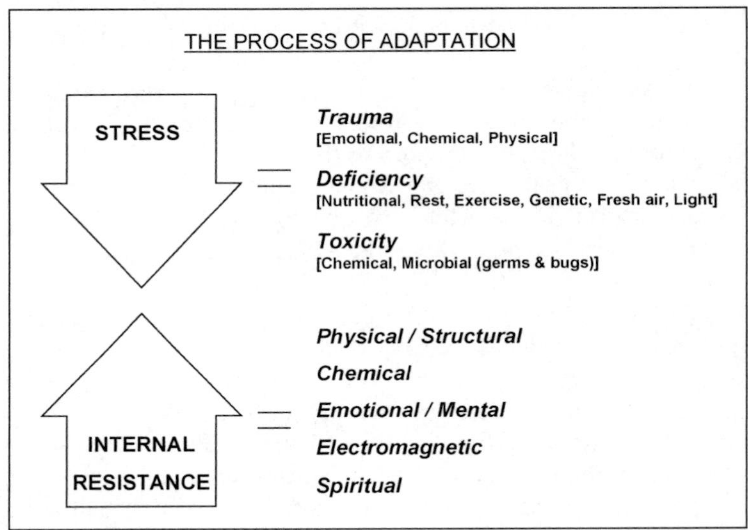

Figure II

Adaptation results from the proper functioning of the body's internal resistance. The greater the resistance, the greater the adaptation. The opposite is also true, the less the resistance, the less the adaptation. Poor adaptation results in dysfunction. Continued dysfunction results in disease.

With low amounts of stress, one would find that the body's internal resistance would be able to process and eliminate toxins, properly digest food, remove waste products and eventually overcome the stress itself with no harmful side effects. This process is constant in everyone.

Moderate amounts of stress require the use of more energy. This degree of adaptation prevents the full expression of health, and will eventually allow for the propagation of disease states and the acceleration of the aging process. Because stress depletes certain nutrients that help keep the immune system strong, those under continual stress usually become worn out or sick. Conditions like asthma, allergies, digestive complaints, headaches, female concerns, pain without any known cause and many more are common. I call these *functional problems* - problems that affect us in some way but don't knock us off our feet. As a protective mechanism, this type of resistance uses low amounts of energy to sustain daily function. It is like driving on the highway in 4th instead of 5th gear. I see this type of patient every day in the office. Their conditions are often self-induced, a result of habit.

As creatures of habit we eat the same foods, go to bed at the same times, engage in the same recreational activities etc. This is fine, if our habits are healthy. If they are not then the body must adapt to the same unhealthy stress over and over again. It is often not until our bodies cry out in pain that we take notice. It is at this point that we must decide whether to make a beneficial change or not.

Severe stress, when your body has been processing multiple stresses for an extended period of time, can be devastating. Because the body cannot keep adapting indefinitely, the regulative processes designed to keep us healthy may accelerate or even backfire. Autoimmune diseases like Rheumatoid Arthritis (RA) and Lupus Erythematosis are good examples. In these patients, the body's own immune system attacks itself creating a debilitating inflammatory process. The inflammatory process is the same in all people. However, in patients with RA or Lupus the mechanism is unchecked and rages out of control. It is a case of the body being unable to regulate a "normal" process. Cancer and other major illnesses can also be included in this category.

The Human Body's Incredible Resistance
Each person's potential resistance is dependent upon their current state of health, genetic make-up and present stress - whatever they are adapting to at the moment. And yet, the same mechanisms are used by each of us to resist all stress.

An incredibly complex defense system has been established throughout the human body. We understand it as our immune system. It is the main form of resistance against various stressors. Up to 70% of the immune system is located in the lining of the intestines. This makes sense since our greatest exposure to the outside world is through the food we eat which may be full of harmful chemicals or bacteria. *People with chronic illnesses and weakened immune systems almost always have digestive complaints at the same time, though it is not fully understood which came first.*

Each of our tissues, when functioning properly, adds to the body's overall resistance. The liver renders toxins harmless; the bowel, kidney and skin wash them away; the heart drives blood flow; muscles encourage lymph drainage; the adrenal glands make all sorts of protective hormones; every cell makes energy; the nervous system transmits messages and on and on.

The ultimate resistance to sickness is through complete functioning. In other words, if the body is given the fuel it needs to run on, processes it completely, eliminates waste, limits exposure to negative stress and experiences growth in the form of positive stress, sickness is rarely an issue. This sounds more complicated than it really is. The opposite however, is also true. If *any* tissue is not functioning well, the body is not as able to resist stress.

The Human Body Is Interconnected
Many Alternative Healthcare Practitioners believe that each of the components of resistance is inter-related and inter-connected to one another. That is to say that any structural problem within the

body, such as a bad back, may very likely have a chemical or even emotional component. I see this very thing on a regular basis in my office. If a patient comes in complaining of upper back pain I will provide the expected structural care: chiropractic adjustments, muscle work, electrical therapy, etc. However, if this problem continues to manifest I will then evaluate the chemical and emotional systems to see if a connection exists. If so, treating this system simultaneously will often produce a profound positive change, much to the patients delight.

The diagram below depicts the three main components the body relies on in order to process and eliminate the stress of bumps, bruises, junk food, worry, fear, anxiety, sleeplessness and any of the other thousand or so stressors present in everyday life.

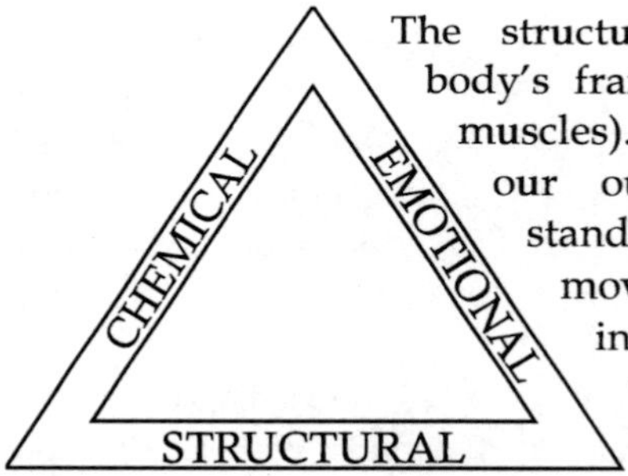

The structural component represents the body's frame and soft tissues (bones and muscles). Our structure is what defines our outward appearance, keeps us standing upright, and allows us to move. The emotional component includes our attitudes and beliefs, while the chemical component consists of the substances needed by our cells, usually received through our diet, the air we breathe and the beverages we drink.

The Human Body Prioritizes Stress

The body has the ability to sacrifice certain tissues for the sake of others. I call this *priority*. This happens through internal mechanisms not fully understood and also because of one's habits. Priority is the reason why two similar people under similar circumstances contract different diseases. Ultimately, genetics may or may not be the primary explanation for priority. Whatever the case, priority is an observable phenomenon and one that makes finding the exact cause of a disease difficult. Priority is also why I do not believe there is such a thing as a wonder drug or single treatment that is able to correct all maladies; some maybe, but not all.

Scoliosis, a progressive disorder of the spine, is a case of an understood priority. No matter how distorted the curves in the spine become, the head will always attempt to keep the eyes parallel with the horizon through a process called the righting reflex. By doing so, the person is best able to function. In other words, it is the body's highest priority to keep the eyes properly oriented. Studying idiopathic diseases (those of unknown origin) and recognizing the priority involved, helps researchers to understand more about the workings of the human body in general. Most of the time however, we determine which tissues the body assigns highest priority to by how we live and the choices we make.

When treating patients with chronic conditions I often notice that the body prioritizes what needs to be fixed. For example, I will check patients for microorganisms, food and chemical sensitivities, heavy metal toxicity and so on. I do so with a specialized technique called applied kinesiology (AK). I discuss this important diagnostic tool at length in the next chapter. On an initial visit I may find microorganisms to be a problem and not find heavy metals. However, after fixing the digestive system and eliminating the harmful microorganisms, heavy metals may now show up. It is as if the body reveals the things that need to be fixed first. It prioritizes. This phenomenon is too common not to be mentioned. The body is simply more complex than we now realize.

Chapter Summary

- The subject of health and disease is controversial, differing among health care providers and influenced by training, upbringing and experience.
- The human body is an infinitely complex creation that exists in a semi-protected state within its environment. It is held together by built-in mechanisms which, although the same, respond and act differently from person to person depending upon their internal resistance and the amount or type of external stress.
- Health is dependent upon the body's ability to not only withstand, but also to overcome constant internal and external stressors.
- If stressors are too great the body adapts – utilizing its reserve capacity.

- When reserves are no longer available imbalances arise and symptoms manifest - indicating a dysfunction within the body.
- The body will make decisions based upon its established priorities.
- Correction of symptoms is accomplished by removing stress in any of its forms, thus relieving part of the overall burden and allowing for the built-in coping mechanisms to focus resources elsewhere.
- Likewise diseases can be overcome by increasing overall resistance. Ideally, both options are pursued. In extreme cases, both are essential.

The above ideas are considered "alternative" and yet are becoming more accepted among healthcare professionals and the public at large.

HEALTH QUESTIONNAIRE

In this chapter I list some of the questions I ask new patients on their first visit. Later, after a course of treatment, I have them answer the same questions. In most cases there is marked improvement. This is a good way to monitor progress.

Use the health questionnaire below to get an idea of your current health status. Keep your results in mind as you read each chapter.

Put a check mark next to the question if the answer is "Yes" or if you currently experience any of the listed symptoms. Count the number of check marks and record them after each section. It is likely that you will need some professional help if in:

- Sections I, II, or III, you checked off five or more questions.
- Section IV (men's total) you checked off ten or more questions.
- Sections IV & V (women's total), you checked off 13 or more questions.

Section I
The following questions relate to adrenal stress and carbohydrate intolerance.

- ❑ Allergies?
- ❑ Always hungry?
- ❑ Anxiety?
- ❑ Asthma?
- ❑ Crave salt?

- ❑ Dizziness upon standing?
- ❑ Drink coffee daily?
- ❑ Fatigue?
- ❑ High blood pressure?
- ❑ Irritable or lightheaded between meals?
- ❑ Leg cramps?
- ❑ Light bothers eyes (always wear sunglasses)?
- ❑ Low blood pressure?
- ❑ Night sweats?
- ❑ Restless legs?
- ❑ Ringing in ears?
- ❑ Sore joints with exercise?
- ❑ Trouble falling asleep?
- ❑ Trouble losing weight even with exercise?
- ❑ Trouble staying asleep?

_______ Total number checked

Section II
The following questions relate to toxicity.

- ❑ Breast tenderness during menstrual cycle?
- ❑ Diarrhea after a fatty meal?
- ❑ Digestive complaints?
- ❑ Eat less than 1 piece of fruit and 2 vegetable servings per day?
- ❑ Eat out more than twice per week?
- ❑ Fatigue?
- ❑ Gallstones?
- ❑ Headaches?
- ❑ High cholesterol?
- ❑ History of Hepatitis?
- ❑ Less than 8 hours of sleep per night?
- ❑ Less than one bowel movement per day?
- ❑ Little or no exercise?
- ❑ More than 3 alcoholic beverages per week?
- ❑ Muscle tenderness without exercise?
- ❑ Often eating meals after 8 p.m.?
- ❑ Often wake up between 2 and 4 a.m.?

- ❑ Pain or swelling in joints?
- ❑ Smoker?
- ❑ Sweat often?

_______ Total number checked

Section III
The following questions relate to a form of intestinal imbalance (dysbiosis) called Candidiasis (see: Common Chronic Conditions).

- ❑ Abdominal bloating after eating?
- ❑ Antibiotic use (this year or more than three times in the last ten years)?
- ❑ Been pregnant?
- ❑ Chemical smells or exposure cause symptoms?
- ❑ Crave alcoholic beverages?
- ❑ Crave breads?
- ❑ Crave sugars?
- ❑ Do you feel worse in humid, damp or moldy places?
- ❑ Ever had prostatitis or vaginitis (itching)?
- ❑ Fungus under finger or toenails?
- ❑ Have taken birth control pills?
- ❑ Have used oral steroids?
- ❑ Frequent skin rashes?
- ❑ Tobacco smoke is very offensive?
- ❑ Vaginal Yeast infections?

_______ Total number checked

Section IV
The following questions relate to general health.

- ❑ 20+ pounds overweight?
- ❑ Abdominal pain?
- ❑ Airline pilot?
- ❑ Arthritis?
- ❑ Cancer?
- ❑ Chest pains?
- ❑ Colitis?

- ❑ Difficulty urinating?
- ❑ Drink less than 4 glasses of water per day?
- ❑ Eat dairy foods most days?
- ❑ Family history of cancer?
- ❑ Family history of diabetes?
- ❑ Family history of heart disease?
- ❑ Family history of mental illness?
- ❑ Family history of stroke?
- ❑ Hemorrhoids?
- ❑ Hospitalized for a non-emergency in the last 12 months?
- ❑ Hospitalized for a non-traumatic emergency in the last 12 months?
- ❑ Long term high or moderate stress?
- ❑ Loss of smell?
- ❑ Loss of taste?
- ❑ Lower back pain?
- ❑ Major lifestyle change (divorce, relocation, loss of job, death of loved one, etc.)?
- ❑ Nasal or sinus congestion?
- ❑ Neck pain?
- ❑ Numbness in toes not related to injury?
- ❑ Pain or swelling in joints?
- ❑ Pins and needles in arms?
- ❑ Sensitive to chemical smells?
- ❑ Serious accident or injury in your lifetime?
- ❑ Shortness of breath?
- ❑ Sick about once per year?
- ❑ Sick more than once per year?
- ❑ Slow healing sores?
- ❑ Sun exposure less than 15 min. per day?
- ❑ Surgery (other)?
- ❑ Surgery as a result of trauma?
- ❑ Surgery on a joint?
- ❑ Surgery on internal organs?
- ❑ Swelling in ankles?
- ❑ Taking more than 2 medications?
- ❑ Visual problems?
- ❑ Work with computers daily?

_______ Total number checked

Section V
(Women Only)

- ❑ Breast tenderness?
- ❑ Constipation?
- ❑ Depression during monthly period?
- ❑ Emotional outbursts?
- ❑ Family history of breast cancer?
- ❑ Headaches around menstrual cycle?
- ❑ Irregular monthly cycles?
- ❑ Menstrual cramping?
- ❑ Oral contraceptive use (past or present)?
- ❑ Under frequent high stress?

_______ Total number checked

APPLIED KINESIOLOGY

The primary purpose of SECTION I, is to make you aware of the numerous ways in which natural medicine can correct and maintain your health. In so doing, I hope to show you that when a health issue arises, you may be better served by seeking natural therapies first rather than traditional medicines.

As described in the chapter, Philosophy, I believe in treating the whole person. This means seeing you as more than sick or broken parts. When a doctor sees your body as many related, non-independent pieces, and treats you as a whole, instead of simply treating a single injured part, the results are most often profound. In fact, many longstanding conditions will simply not resolve without a whole-person approach (see: SECTION II: Common Chronic Conditions).

There are many natural health clinics that specialize in different techniques: acupuncture, chiropractic, muscle therapy, nutrition and so on. Each of these therapies, in and of themselves, can be powerful and effective at restoring proper bodily function. Unfortunately, no therapy is a panacea - each has its limits. At times a patient requires more of one kind of therapy than another. And yet, if these therapies are used in combination, as is commonly so in my office, the benefit for the patient can then be exponential. The challenge is knowing which therapy to use at which time. The answer is found in a diagnostic system called applied kinesiology. I have chosen to discuss applied kinesiology first for the simple reason that, when used appropriately, it can be the most effective form of diagnosis for functional illness.

Applied kinesiology (A.K.) is a natural health care system based on an evaluation of the body's structural, biochemical and mental aspects. A.K. primarily uses muscle testing to augment other standard methods of diagnosis. A.K. is now used by many health-care professionals including chiropractors, medical doctors, osteopaths and dentists.

Background

Applied kinesiology began in 1964 through the work of its founder George Goodheart, D.C. Today, a governing body called the International College of Applied Kinesiology (I.C.A.K) determines and defines what is and what is not A.K. Members of the I.C.A.K., who include chiropractors, medical doctors, osteopaths, dentists and more, must adhere to these rules and regulations, in order to be given appropriate status within the college. It is the goal of the I.C.A.K. to present its diagnostic and treatment techniques to the critical medical mainstream as a viable adjunct or alternative to existing health care. This can only be done with solid scientific evidence. Despite the lack of funding for research into alternative medical approaches the scientific support for Applied Kinesiology is growing. Numerous articles have been published in peer-reviewed literature, with several other research studies awaiting publication. A host of articles related to other forms of alternative health care may also be cited as support for the philosophy and practice of A.K.

What Is Muscle Testing?

Muscle testing is a functional neurological assessment. An A.K. doctor can evaluate the muscles of the body and gain some understanding of a patient's overall health. For instance, it has been known for centuries that specific muscles have relationships to specific organs. It has been discovered in the last several decades that every muscle is in some way related to an organ. When an organ is not functioning properly it may cause a disruption in the muscle group with which it is associated. This interference is called a viscero-somatic reflex. The opposite is also true. If a muscle is injured it can negatively affect the function of an organ – a somato-visceral reflex. For example, the quadriceps muscle on the front of the thigh is related to the small intestine. It is quite possible for an individual with a duodenal ulcer, when tested properly, to be found to have less than optimum function of their quadriceps muscle. The deltoids, the muscles closely related to the lungs, are another example. Almost all asthma patients have one or more weak shoulder muscles. Treating weak muscles and making them stronger by the structural, chemical or emotional tools of A.K. has been shown to have a significant impact on the related organ system as well.

What Makes Muscle Testing So Special?

Simply fixing weak muscles is just the beginning with A.K. The fascinating thing about muscle testing is what happens when the nervous system is exposed to different stimuli. A change in a muscle test (i.e. from strong to weak or weak to strong) may be noticed with the introduction or removal of a given stimuli, such as: chemicals, smells, pressure, touch, temperature, thoughts, electromagnetic fields or anything else that may be processed by the nervous system. When performed correctly, a change in muscle function may be noticed, with even the slightest stimuli. These changes are immediate and may occur with or without a disease present. This means that a non-serious (functional) problem can be discovered prior to its becoming serious, a boast made by few other diagnostics methods.

What Is The Meaning Of A Muscle Test?

Generally speaking, stimuli that will have a positive effect on the patient will strengthen muscles that originally test weak, and stimuli that will have an adverse effect on the patient will weaken muscles that originally test strong. However, it is impossible and improper to emphatically state the meaning of a given muscle test alone. A weak muscle test by itself only tells the doctor that something is wrong. Muscle testing does not tell the doctor why something is wrong. Many variables are present in the overall picture of a patient's health. A detailed history, consultation, examination, and traditional diagnostic testing must be combined with muscle testing in order to formulate a proper plan of treatment.

Is Muscle Testing An Accepted Practice In Medicine?

Not yet. Muscle testing is quite controversial for a few good reasons. On a theoretical level, as with most alternative health care practices, some of the technique's foundational ideas and its unorthodox approach are hard for the medically trained mind to understand. On a practical level, it seems too good to be true. Are changes in muscle response possible by merely touching, tasting or even thinking? Skeptics would say no, suggesting that the doctor is somehow influencing the test results. We have no problem with the doubts of outside observers. It is normal to question what one doesn't understand. However, for the skeptic, all that is required is a closer look. Consider for instance one of the most controversial aspects within A.K., oral nutrient testing.

A doctor may place a chemical or food in the patient's mouth and then test to see if a strong muscle becomes weak. This idea is preposterous to the traditional medical mind. However, from a neurological standpoint this response is entirely possible. The pathway from the nerve endings on the tongue to the brain and then back out to the testing muscle is clearly understood. Also, since electricity travels at the speed of light, and the messages within and from the brain are transmitted electrically, there should be no problem accepting the seemingly instant change of a muscle's strength when a substance is tasted. In fact, it is known that the nervous system is able to process *10^{13} bits of information per second* in the unconscious mind. Equipped with this information, the sincere skeptic should recognize the plausibility of what has been stated.

Correcting an Imbalance

Remember the last time you bumped your elbow against the wall or the corner of a counter top? The first thing you probably did was to touch and rub the painful spot. Rubbing actually made the pain more bearable or it may have taken it away altogether. There is a very good reason for this. It is well known in neurology that different nerve endings or sensory receptors (like touch and pressure receptors) have different priorities in the nervous system. Mechanical stimulation such as rubbing has a high priority in the brain and will "cover up" any other sensations such as pain. So when you rub your elbow, in essence you are making your brain pay more attention to the sensation of touch and pressure than to the sensation of pain. An A.K. doctor uses muscle testing to determine which sensory information will produce a therapeutic effect. Then by adding the right sensory information in the right manner a favorable outcome is most often achieved.

Once a stimulus is found that strengthens a weak muscle, that stimulus can be introduced in greater measure producing a therapeutic response. In the case above, rubbing your elbow was therapeutic for reducing pain. The same is true for nutritional or chemical stimulation. If a weak muscle became strong after having the patient taste a vitamin C tablet, this may indicate that their body has a need for vitamin C. Any stimulus that produces a weakness in a previously strong muscle should be further evaluated to see if it may be contributing to the cause of a patient's dysfunction.

When testing muscles using A.K. if a muscle tests weak, this does not usually mean that exercises are required. The weakness found is often neurological. In other words, for a variety of reasons, muscle are sometimes shut off or "turned down."

The turning on and turning off of muscles happens every time you move. In order to walk you must contract the muscles in the front of the leg while at the same time relaxing the muscles on the back of the leg. If this were not so your muscles would contract at the same time and your leg would not move. The process of turning on one group of muscles while the opposite, or antagonist muscle group stays relaxed, is called *reciprocal inhibition*. This process happens subconsciously. There are other unconscious processes that shut off or turn on muscles in order to prevent injury.

In the middle of any muscle group are sensory cells called spindle cells. These cells automatically contract a muscle whenever it is stretched too far. Another set of cells located where the muscle attaches to the bone are called Golgi tendon organs. These cells automatically relax a muscle whenever it is over-contracted.
Treatments to help muscles regain function will often require precise stimulation of either or both of these cell groups.

If a patient injures their lower back, I will check all of the muscles around the hips, pelvis and spine. I will nearly always find one or more muscles that do not test strong; they have been automatically turned off by the body as a protective measure. I will then stimulate the cells in the belly of the muscle or at the attachment sites of the muscle and retest to see if the muscle strengthens. If so, more therapy is continued at the site that produced strength.

Below is a summary of three other techniques that can be used to help weak muscles return to their intended strength. In order to be fully appreciated more detail is required beyond the scope of this book.

- *Neurolymphatic Reflex Stimulation* – These reflexes are located throughout the trunk and extremities. They relate to both a particular muscle and a particular organ (i.e. thigh muscles relate to the small intestine). Stimulating these reflexes with gentle circular pressure often produces a dramatic increase in the function of the related muscle and organ.
- *Neurovascular Reflex Stimulation* – Like neurolymphatic reflexes that have both a muscle and an organ related to them, neurovascular reflexes have similar relationships but are located on the head. Light sustained pressure is all that is required to stimulate these reflexes and produce a therapeutic effect.
- *Injury Recall Technique (IRT)* – When a tissue is injured, the body places a high priority on its healing. Also, all sorts of chemical and neurological processes begin. During the healing process the tissue will be in a state of reduced function and will likely be painful or sensitive to touch. That is because the sensory nerves located around and within the tissue are on high alert. This state reminds the rest of the body that this area is under repair. The nerves will maintain their state of heightened sensitivity until complete healing has occurred. Sometimes, for whatever reason, this does not take place, and so tissue function is reduced and the nerves remain highly sensitive. When present, a deeper neurological therapy is required in order for proper function to be restored.

  The procedure is very simple, but often produces a surprisingly strong therapeutic response. Two steps are required. 1. The doctor stimulates the previously injured area - usually with gentle pinching. 2. The doctor then immediately applies gentle downward pressure on a bone in the foot called the talus. That's it!

  The neurological explanation for the effectiveness of this treatment is somewhat complicated and has to do with all of the sensory nerves located throughout the foot. The messages from these nerves are given a high priority in the brain because they are responsible for keeping us upright and oriented when we stand on our feet. Somehow, stimulating a previously injured area and then immediately stimulating the sensory receptors in the foot, produces a reduction in nerve sensitivity and an increase in function of the previously injured tissue.

One of my patients had a return of normal vision as a result IRT. She was struck in the head with a discus many years prior, and gradually her eyesight worsened. I performed this simple procedure on the scarred area where the impact occurred and her vision returned to normal within fifteen minutes. This response is in no way typical but it does demonstrate that subtle neurologically based therapies can have dramatic results.

In summary, correction of an imbalance discovered through A.K. testing of the patient's structural, chemical or emotional health is achieved through a myriad of therapies including chiropractic adjustments, cranial bone alignment, neurolymphatic correction and neurovascular stimulation, acupressure, nutritional supplementation and more. In other words, A.K. helps to find the problem, and often determines the appropriate form of treatment needed to correct it.

Factors That Influence the Outcome of a Muscle Test

Theoretically, patients with many health problems should be good candidates for muscle testing. In fact, the opposite may be true. Their bodies spend so much time adapting to, and correcting existing imbalances, that additional stimuli introduced by the doctor (like checking for a subluxation or an allergy) produce little or no change whatsoever in a muscle test. It is like trying to hear a whisper in a crowded room. Any of the following factors may be a significant hindrance to muscle testing:

- Cigarette smoking.
- Poor diet.
- Obesity.
- Many major chronic illnesses.

- Poor bioelectric conduction – how cells communicate electrically.
- Severe chemical, structural or emotional stress.

Because of the problems above, techniques have been developed to "clear" a patient before attempting to derive any significant information from muscle tests. In my experience I clear a patient by evaluating their neurological function. This can be done by simply having the patient simulate walking while lying on their back. This activity, called cross-crawl, activates the right and left sides of the brain. To evaluate further, I also have the patient contact two known neurological points on their upper sternum. While touching these points the patient breathes deeply as I look for certain changes in structural balance and position. This test evaluates the communication between the body and the brain. Checking for and correcting both of these important areas only takes a few minutes. If these two tests are not responding properly, then muscle testing results may be inaccurate.

What Are The Limitations of Applied Kinesiology?

It is important to note that the overall skill level of the doctor using A.K. muscle testing is dependent upon many factors: knowledge of nutrition, physiology, neurochemistry and sensory receptor-based therapies as well as doctor consistency and experience. Unfortunately there are many health care professionals who say they are using Applied Kinesiology, but in fact are not. These doctors may be using muscle testing and its associated terminology, but their particular technique cannot be found in the official teaching of the I.C.A.K. To ensure that you are getting a qualified doctor, ask if they if they have undergone the necessary training given by the I.C.A.K.

Conclusion

Applied Kinesiology is an extremely beneficial tool in the hands of a doctor who understands its strengths and weaknesses. Working on the more sensitive functional level, A.K. can help to identify dysfunction or potential disease prior to its appearance through the evaluation of the body's three main physical components: structural, chemical and emotional/mental. Currently, A.K. is the only known form of diagnosis, alternative or conventional, with this capability. The technique is both a science and an art, and, like other health procedures, is not perfect. A.K. therefore is used in conjunction with other recognized forms of diagnosis and treatment.

It is my strong belief that even with its current lack of full recognition, applied kinesiology will continue to grow, becoming more recognized and further incorporated into other forms of medicine.

STRUCTURAL THERAPIES

Bones, muscles, ligaments, tendons and other soft tissues make up the structure of the body. These tissues can be kept healthy through a variety of techniques – some of which are discussed in this book.

Structural care is the primary concern for most chiropractors, physical therapists, massage therapists and personal trainers. However, as you will learn by reading this information, structural complaints are many times the result of underlying chemical and even emotional stresses.

Most patients seek out structural care for orthopedic conditions such as:

- Neck Pain
- Lower Back Pain
- Shoulder or extremity pain
- Muscle pain
- Headaches

Described below are the techniques I use to correct structural problems. These techniques are non-invasive, low-force, and very effective.

SPINAL ADJUSTMENTS

In chiropractic college students are bombarded daily with the philosophy of spinal wellness. They are taught that there is a direct relationship between a properly aligned spinal column and good health. These ideas are all true. Spinal adjustments are part of every treatment I perform whether correcting migraines, food allergies, colitis, a hiatal hernia or anything else.

A spinal adjustment is designed to eliminate what chiropractors call, a subluxation. This is a fancy name for an improperly positioned spinal bone (vertebra). Subluxations are often areas of pain, discomfort and swelling. They require attention because their presence in the spine usually means that something else is wrong with the body.

There are a number of ways to correct subluxated bones. I have chosen techniques that use very low force. This means that you will typically not hear "popping" or "cracking" with an adjustment. Low-force adjustments are extremely effective at restoring normal function to the spine or other boney structures.

Each segment of the spine is directly related to different organs by the nerves that connect them. There are many indirect connections through the muscular and electrical systems as well. Chemical toxicity, tissue strain or sprain, muscle imbalances from excess work, poor posture, and even emotional stress may eventually produce a subluxation in the related area of the spine. In fact, any stress is capable of creating a subluxation.

Correcting subluxations often has a profound effect on the tissues under stress. That is why it is not uncommon for a chiropractor to correct a seemingly unrelated problem like asthma or menstrual cramps simply by performing spinal adjustments.

A patient came into the office for a recurring problem in the middle of his back. Three or four times over the course of six weeks, he would need to be "put back in place." After further investigation however, it was discovered that because his adrenal glands were under significant stress, he was sensitive to the hormone insulin. After treating him for this problem alone, he no longer needed to be adjusted in his mid-back.

In this case, a subluxation resulted from an insulin imbalance. What's more, most insulin imbalances result from ingesting too many carbohydrates. In other words, it is quite possible that eating spaghetti and bread sticks – one of his favorites - caused the pain in his back!

Chiropractic adjustments are one of the healthiest things you can do for yourself, but they are not a cure-all. As stated previously, subluxations are often secondary to organ or tissue stress. If the primary issue is not addressed, subluxations will have a tendency to recur. As you will discover, we use a number of techniques to evaluate and correct the primary cause of a subluxation – not just the subluxation itself. Because of the potential benefits, it is important to regularly seek care for your spine and all other tissues. This often means a short visit every month or so. Consider this: Dentists rightly suggest our need for regular check-ups. If regular check-ups are good for teeth (which have one function) how important are they for a multi-purpose spine that carries the lifeline of the body?

VECTOR POINT CRANIAL THERAPY

Vector point cranial therapy is the primary method I use for correcting spinal subluxations. This therapy is low force and non-invasive. Vector point cranial therapy operates from the premise that most of the subluxations in the body are secondary to a primary subluxation. Once the primary subluxation is corrected, any secondary subluxation will correct on its own. Primary subluxations are located in either the cranium or pelvis. All other subluxations are compensatory and may be located throughout the spine or the jaw. One of the main components of cranium and pelvis subluxations is something called dural tension.

The dura is a fibrous sheet that covers the brain and spinal cord. Its attachments begin inside the skull and then work their way down the spinal canal, finally anchoring at the lowest bone in the spine, the sacrum. It has many purposes, one of which is to allow for the free flowing of cerebral spinal fluid. This process, called the Cranial Sacral Respiratory Mechanism, is maintained in part by the subtle movements of the cranial bones.

When the cranial bones are subluxated dural tension is created. When dural tension is created, the uppermost neck vertebrae and the jaw joints react. When the uppermost vertebrae react, the rest of the body, including soft tissues like organs, adapt. From one subluxation, an entire pattern of compensation and adaptation takes place within the body.

How It Works

By applying sustained gentle pressure to the cranium on specific points we are able to gradually move the cranial bones back into their original position. Because this process also removes dural tension, the net effect is not only the correction of the cranial bones themselves, but also the correction of all other secondary distortions of the spine. Usually three or four points must be contacted simultaneously in order to properly reposition the cranial bones. The procedure is enhanced by having the patient breath deeply while flexing their feet. Movement of the feet and toes upward while inhaling slightly stretches the dura while moving the feet and toes downward while exhaling relaxes the dura.

Patients welcome Vector Point Cranial Therapy as a substitute for more traditional forms of spinal adjustments, which generally require high levels of force. They are also pleasantly surprised that such a subtle technique can have so profound an effect. When the mechanisms of spinal distortions are understood, it soon becomes clear that the success of Vector Point Cranial Therapy lies in both the precision of the treatment itself and in the skill of the doctor performing the treatment.

CRANIAL SACRAL THERAPY

One of the most powerful techniques for correcting a myriad of health problems is also one of the most subtle. Cranial Sacral Therapy is a gentle, low-force adjustive technique that works primarily on the bones of the skull.

The Skull

It has long been believed that the sole purpose of the skull was to protect the brain. While this role is obviously paramount, research has shown that the skull has other important functions. The skull bones actually move as with breathing. There are eight major joints within the skull called sutures. Sutures act like hinges on which the cranial bones move as you inhale and exhale. The movement is minute and is not seen with the naked eye. The synchronous movement of the cranial bones is necessary for proper function of the spine, nervous and energy systems. It is believed that the primary reason for the movement of the cranial bones is for distribution of cerebral spinal fluid, which flows outside of the brain and the spinal cord. The body can make up to several liters of this fluid per day. Misalignments of the cranial bones are called cranial faults. Some of the more common symptoms of cranial faults are:

- Headaches
- Migraines
- Sinus problems
- Neck problems
- Visual disturbances

There are other symptoms as well. Since cranial bone movement effects nerve and energy patterns throughout the body, it is possible for almost any symptom to be the result of a cranial fault.

Cranial faults may develop for a variety of reasons. Many professionals believe that primary cranial faults are the result of birth trauma or trauma sometime in the development of the child before the skull bones were fully formed. In my experience, I commonly see cranial faults as a result of chemical (nutritional) or even emotional trauma as well. This means that a poor diet or a stressful event can produce cranial faults as much as a car accident or a fall. That is why I always attempt to evaluate the whole person.

Finding Cranial Faults

A simple way that I test for cranial faults is by looking for changes in leg length while the patient breaths deeply. Breathing is a good way to look for cranial faults because the cranial bones move with each phase of respiration. If they are subluxated (not moving properly) there will be other recognizable changes throughout the body.

Before beginning, I examine the patient while they are lying on their back, looking to see if their feet are even at the heels or if there is a discrepancy from one side to the other. It is common for people to have uneven leg lengths when evaluated in this way. I then have the patient breath in and out deeply. If there is a change in the measurement of the feet, then I know that cranial faults are present. The cranial bones may also be evaluated through muscle testing as part of an applied kinesiological examination. If there are cranial faults, gentle pressure to the bones of the head, applied in a specific direction, will cause a strong muscle to temporarily weaken. Correction is made with gentle pressure as the patient breaths. Patients are generally surprised at the effectiveness of this technique and often describe immediate relief following cranial therapy. They are also surprised to discover that the body behaves so dynamically with even small amounts of stimulus. It is because of these dynamic changes that we are able to correct many conditions with low or non-forceful techniques.

EXERCISE PROGRAMS

Exercise is one of the most important things you can do to obtain and maintain health. However, all exercises are not created equal. The type of exercise you engage in is very important. Most of my patients are initially put on an aerobic building program. The details of this program are discussed in SECTION III. Below is a summary of the benefits of aerobic training.

Aerobic System
Aerobic training, (light jogging, easy swimming, easy biking etc.), uses oxygen to burn fat, and is best engaged by prolonged steady use of the slow muscle fibers in our legs. The body is designed to burn fat as its primary fuel, but this is not always the case. As life's stresses increase, the human metabolism begins burning more sugar creating disrupted hormonal patterns. My program is designed to return the body to a primarily fat-burning metabolism.

The same amount of fat contains more than twice as much potential fuel as carbohydrates. In order to engage this system and burn fat, exercise must occur within a low heart rate range.

Walking and other forms of aerobic exercise have been recommended for all people, because of their health promoting effects.

Benefits of aerobic exercise:

- Increases blood circulation to all tissues.
- Increases energy levels.
- Strengthens immune system.
- Promotes fat loss.
- Detoxifies tissues and eliminates waste.
- Decreases stress on sensitive tissues like the adrenal glands.

- Reduces the chance of over-training.

There are many specifics that must be addressed concerning proper exercise. Please see: SECTION III: Exercise, for more detailed information.

ORTHOPEDIC SUPPORTS

ORTHOTICS

Your feet are the foundation of your body. They support you when you stand, walk, or run. They also help protect your entire body from damaging stress as you move around. Your feet perform best when all their muscles, arches and bones are in their ideal stable positions. Any weakness or unstable positioning in the feet often contributes to postural problems in the rest of the body, which may lead to spinal misalignment.

A common problem is for the arch of the foot to drop, causing pronation, or a rolling inward of the ankle. When this occurs the knee also becomes unstable and consequently so does the pelvis and lower back. An unstable foot could cause a host of painful conditions. In these cases I often recommend custom-made spinal/pelvic stabilizers, commonly called orthotics, to my patients. They help to support the arch, reduce pain and contribute to your total body wellness. They also help your spinal adjustments last longer.

You are a unique individual – no one else is exactly like you. The same goes for your feet. Custom-made, prescription stabilizers are crafted from a mold of your foot that is made in the office. The mold is then sent to the manufacturer along with any additional information your doctor may discover upon examination so that, once created, your stabilizer is perfectly tailored.

To see if orthotics are required I often use a simple muscle test. While the patient is standing in a relaxed position, I test the strength of an arm muscle. Usually it is strong. Then I have the patient roll their feet inward, placing stress on the arch of the foot. While maintaining this position, I retest the same strong muscle. I then have the patient roll their feet outward and retest the strong muscle. If in either of these positions the strong muscle becomes weak, I know that some sort of problem is present in the feet or ankles. I then have the patient stand on an orthotic and repeat the procedure above. If this time their arm muscle remains strong, an orthotic will probably help.

NECK SUPPORT – CERVICAL PILLOWS

Patients often ask for advice regarding their mattress and pillows, knowing intuitively that poor spinal support while sleeping is detrimental to their structure. In fact, sleeping in an improper position is a common cause of pain in the lower back and neck.

Sometimes patients complain of neck pain that is quickly corrected in the office, only to call the next morning to report that the pain had returned. Most likely in these instances, the patient is sleeping with the wrong kind of pillow. The right pillow will relieve aches and pains as well as improve your sleep quality.

Again, as in the case of the orthotics, I use applied kinesiology to help me determine if a cervical pillow is required. While the patient lies on their back on the treatment table I check for a strong leg muscle. I then change the type of pillow under their head and retest the same strong muscle looking for a weakness. If a weakness is produced, that pillow is not right for the patient. Pillows of varying heights are placed under the head and the strong leg muscle is tested. I then have the patient change position to their side and check the same pillows again. Through a process of elimination I will arrive at a pillow that works in all sleeping positions for this particular patient.

Other indicators are often used at the same time. For instance, I can probe the neck for any areas of tenderness. When the patient rests on a pillow that inappropriate for their needs, the area of tenderness will stay just as tender, or in many cases, get worse. However, when resting on an appropriate pillow – one that does not cause a weakness of a strong leg muscle - the tenderness of the area in the neck is often greatly reduced.

NUTRITIONAL THERAPIES

Every second, thousands of chemical and metabolic processes take place within our cells and tissues. Thinking, breathing, detoxifying, digesting and all other bodily processes require specific types and amounts of nutrients in order to function properly. Knowing this, it is easy to understand how deficiencies in the quality and quantity of nutrients will lead to dysfunction. At best, deficiencies result in poor function that is easily corrected; at worst they lead to malfunctioning - more commonly know as disease. In fact, every top-ten killer in America is directly or indirectly related to nutritional deficiencies.

Healing is a process that requires proper nutrients; therefore virtually any condition that a patient suffers from is bound to call for a nutritional component to enhance their recovery. This is why I commonly use nutrients to help patients with what seem to be primary structural problems like a sprained ankle or a sore back. There are also certain conditions for which nutritional therapy becomes paramount to the health of the patient such as in the case of allergies and toxicity from a poor diet.

DIET

The human body is made up of countless numbers of chemicals, each designed to carry out a specific function for the benefit of the body as a whole. The presence of essential chemicals means a better chance for vibrant health, while the absence of essential chemicals means a better chance for disease. This is important for our discussion on diet because the nutrients (chemicals) we require for health can only come from what we eat.

When the cells of our body die and new cells are formed, the material needed to make those tissues comes from the macro and micronutrients in our diet. Macronutrients include three main building blocks: carbohydrates, proteins and fats. The micronutrients include: minerals, vitamins, enzymes and thousands of other co-factors whose job it is to regulate the activity of the macronutrients. What this means is that a poor diet results in poor nutrition and creates a greater potential for disease.

Of all the erroneous ideas believed and taught in the health field, none is as shocking or hazardous as the belief that diet has little to do with the prevention or elimination of disease. Thankfully this idea is slowly dying out. Science repeatedly confirms what most of us have known all along: good diets make you healthy, while bad diets eventually cause illness.

I regularly use diet modification and nutritional measures to greatly relieve or eliminate chronic ailments. The guidelines I use are easy to understand and follow.

Another Diet?

There are dozens of available diets to pick and choose from in the marketplace. Each claims that it is the right one for you. However, it is important to remember that people are not all the same. The physical condition a person finds himself in today is the result of their genetics, life events and the choices they have made throughout their lifetime. No two people have the same genetic makeup, and no two people have had the same experiences. This means that it is highly unlikely that a single diet will be able to meet the needs of all people. In our office we use many different diets to help restore health, including:

- Body Type Diet
- Blood Type Diet
- High Protein Diet
- Detoxification Diet
- Yeast Avoidance Diet (see: Candida, in Common Chronic Conditions)

After having made good progress on their prescribed diet listed above, patients are transitioned to the Maintenance Diet. The Maintenance Diet is nothing more than sound eating principles with some variation depending on a patient's individual needs. I discuss the Maintenance Diet in SECTION III: Diet & Food.

SUPPLEMENTATION

According to the United States Department of Agriculture (USDA), more than 70 percent of men and women eat less than two-thirds of the Recommended Daily Intake (RDI) for one or more nutrients. Only 10 percent of the American population eats five or more servings of fruits and vegetables per day. In other words, the standard American diet is rich in low-nutrient, fatty foods comprised of empty calories and little nutritional value.

Vitamins and minerals play essential roles in all body processes including proper growth, digestion, energy production, hormone synthesis and regulation, immune system function, detoxification, nerve and muscle function, and reproduction.

Supplementation can be one of the most effective treatments for any health condition. It is well known that certain diseases are directly related to improper amounts of vitamins: Scurvy – Vitamin C; Beriberi – Vitamin B1; Pellagra – Vitamin B3; Rickets – Vitamin D, and so on. It is my firm belief that *all* illnesses have a nutritional component. This makes perfect sense because every process in the body is dependent upon proper nutrition. Since I work in the functional realm – the area between health and identifiable disease – I see daily, the profound negative effects resulting from even mild nutritional deficiencies, and the power of proper supplementation to reverse those effects.

With the growth of the Vitamin/Supplement industry and their massive advertising campaigns, public awareness of the need for vitamins and minerals is increasing. It is not surprising then to find that most people are taking some form of supplementation. Usually they have read in a magazine or heard from a friend that a certain supplement is good for a particular condition. Others realize that their diets are less than optimal and therefore do the prudent thing by boosting nutrition in the form of a one-per-day multiple vitamins. I agree that nutritional supplements are important and applaud the enthusiasm and willingness of people who take the necessary steps to improve their health.

Unfortunately, most are not getting what they need from their supplements for a variety of reasons.

When supplements don't work

When patients are tested with Applied Kinesiology for the effectiveness of their supplements, I often find that a striking number do very little; some are detrimental to a certain tissue, while others are in fact toxic. Many products simply do not work either because of poor quality, added preservative agents designed to extend shelf life, or the improper combining of essential nutrients. Also, high quality is not always enough.

It is not uncommon for new patients to arrive at the office carrying a bag filled with several dozen supplements. They have heard the latest report about this or that "wonder" herb, and then on their own purchased it from the health food store. The herb may in fact be beneficial but there is a problem. Every person is metabolically specific. This means that supplements that work for one person may not work for others. One's metabolism is also very dynamic. It changes rapidly in some cases based on diet, stress, lack of rest, increased or decreased activity and more. This adds to the confusion concerning which supplements to take, because it may mean that the ones that worked so well for so long are now not effective. For these reasons we often ask the patient to bring in their supplements for testing and then retest those same supplements at a later date.

Treating with Supplements

Supplements can be used in a variety of ways to help restore proper function. The degree to which an imbalance is present determines how much of a given supplement the patient needs. For example, if a patient shows a great need for vitamin B1, giving them a multi-vitamin that contains B1 will not do. *An imbalance must be treated with an imbalance.* This means that we must supplement with a *high level* of B1 for a period of time and then recheck those levels at a later date to make sure everything is in balance. Rechecking regularly for any supplement that a patient takes is important because what was good for them in the past may not be good for them in the present. The body will only improve and stay healthy when it is given the correct supplements in their correct amounts.

DETOXIFICATION

Detoxification is simply a term that means to get rid of toxins. It is perhaps the most essential practice of any health care regime. Detoxification is so important a process that most of our tissues participate in it, and all of our tissues are dependent upon it. Everyone needs to detoxify. Below I describe some general information regarding the topic. Additional information is found in SECTION III: Detoxification.

Contraindications:
Although everyone needs to detoxify, some people need special consideration and should consult with a doctor knowledgeable in nutrition and detoxification protocols before starting:

- Obese persons
- Women who are pregnant
- Nursing moms
- Persons with diabetes
- Persons with hypoglycemia
- Persons with insulin insensitivity
- Persons with intestinal yeast
- Persons with all forms of irritable bowel disease

How Do I Become Toxic?
Today we are exposed to more chemicals and pollutants than in any previous generation. For example, according to the book, An Alternative Medicine Definitive Guide To Cancer, "70 million Americans live in areas that exceed smog standards; most municipal drinking water contains over 700 chemicals, including excessive levels of lead. Some 3,000 chemicals are added to the food supply and as many as 10,000 chemicals, in the form of solvents, emulsifiers, and preservatives, are used in food processing and storage, which can remain in the body for years."

The reason toxins are stored is a matter of efficiency. Though the resources within our bodies allocated for detoxification are numerous and redundant, they are still finite. If more toxins come in to the body than can be processed at any given moment, then the body must store them. Storing toxins is much less harmful than allowing them to float freely in our blood. Usually fat and muscle are the storage tissues of choice. Eventually however, if this toxin accumulation continues, the immune system suffers and the body will manifest the symptoms of toxicity.

What Should I Expect?

Detoxification is not fun and is often not easy. When done incorrectly, the experience can be downright awful. If the detoxification tissues are not ready to process and eliminate, you may feel or even become ill. Headaches, nausea, dizziness, colds, and other less than desirable symptoms are all possible during detoxification. You may ask, "If detoxification is so bad, why do it?" We have to remember something very important: Toxins are powerful and harmful. They are poisons. The body did the right thing by storing them but it makes no sense to keep them around any longer. The prudent thing to do is to get rid of them in the least uncomfortable and most effective way.

I use a number of helpful nutrients and suggestions to enhance your detoxification program. In fact, anything you do to make yourself healthier will also encourage detoxification.

Components

Just like controlling stress, detoxification is improved in one of two ways: reduce the number of toxins coming in, and/or increase your body's ability to remove toxins by improving the function of the detoxification tissues. Below is a list of possible recommendations for your individual detoxification program.

REMOVE TOXINS:	*INCREASE FUNCTION:*
Diet	Exercise/ Massage
Stress Reduction	Colon Cleanse
Supplementation	Liver Cleanse
Water Purification	Kidney Cleanse
Air Purification	Skin Brushing
	Fasting

Figure III

The best detoxification program would incorporate as many of the above as possible. Some should be done daily for a short time period, while others should be done forever. *For most, detoxification should be an annual or semi-annual routine.*

EMOTIONAL THERAPIES

The chapter on Philosophy described the human body as a triangle where each side directly influences the other two. The structural, chemical and emotional components make up the three sides of the triangle. Each of these components is vital to health.

I use diet and nutritional supplementation to help the chemical aspects, exercise and hands-on therapies to help the structural aspects, and a technique called N.E.T. to help with the emotional aspects. This description however, is somewhat simplistic. As you have already discovered, it is nearly impossible to isolate one aspect of the body. In other words, when a doctor corrects a structural problem, he also changes a patient's chemistry, which in turn, influences the patient's emotional health. This is why it is possible to help emotional problems by treating the spine, muscles, or other reflex points on the body.

NEURO-EMOTIONAL THERAPY (N.E.T)

It is human nature to have an emotional response to significant events in our lives and then return to our "normal" state of being after the body has properly processed the event. Sometimes however, because of some form of physiological deficit, the body is unable to fully process an emotional response, so it stores or "locks" it in our nervous system. Storing emotional responses is one way in which the body copes with extreme stress. This phenomenon is called a neuro-emotional complex (N.E.C.). Eventually, an N.E.C. may cause imbalances in structure or chemistry. This means that a patient may have pain, food intolerances, or any number of symptoms as a result of a previously stored emotional event.

I use muscle testing, body reflex points, and semantic reactions (physiologic reactions to memories or words) to help the patient recall any negative events that may be part of a neuro-emotional complex. Once found, certain details of the negative emotional event are assessed. For instance, if a patient experiences a great deal of fear, it is often helpful to pinpoint the origin of the fear. This is usually an event some time in their past. The original fearful event makes it difficult for later fearful events to be properly processed. Therefore, correcting the memory of the original event is not only helpful for that specific N.E.C. but also for other similar emotional events.

The N.E.T. Correction

After the Neuro-Emotional Complex is found I am ready to begin treatment. While the patient maintains the thought of the emotional event, I treat whatever areas of the spine become misaligned, or subluxated (for more information about subluxations see the article on spinal adjustments). I may also treat acupressure points, reflex points or a host of other areas in order balance the body and remove the N.E.C.

What Else You Need To Know

- N.E.T is painless, non-invasive and very safe.
- N.E.T does not take the place of professional counseling but is instead a complimentary part of any healthcare procedure focused on treating the *entire person*. Patients who show a need for psychotherapy are referred to a qualified professional.
- Although N.E.T. procedures are non-complex, their therapeutic effect is profound. Often patients will comment that they feel an immediate relief.
- N.E.T does not deal with the spiritual realm.
- N.E.T. does not make claims about the past. Some N.E.C.s may have actually happened in the past. Others may be associated with imagined emotional events, such as nightmares, or misperceptions. Recalled events are termed

"emotional reality," because they may or may not correspond with actual historical reality.

Emotional stresses are powerful. Fortunately, through the use of N.E.T we have an effective means of overcoming these obstacles to health.

ENERGETIC THERAPIES

In your daily life a dynamic energy exchange is occurring between you, others and the outside world. This exchange is the combination of mental, emotional and physical energies, not all of which are health-promoting. The topic of subtle energies like the negative emotions of the people around you or the presence of electromagnetic fields, are somewhat controversial because they are not fully understood. They should however, be taken seriously.

There are an ever-increasing number of electromagnetic sources such as electrical appliances, computers, cell phones, microwaves, air planes, and fluorescent lights. It is known that prolonged exposure to these electromagnetic fields does negatively impact the health of the human body. Because of these facts, it is likely that illnesses caused by the stress of electromagnetic fields will, in the near future, become one of the primary reasons for seeking care from a physician.

Electromagnetic fields (EMFs) range from Gamma and X-rays which have a very high frequency (1022 Hz) down to 60 Hertz household electricity and even lower. They are measured in a unit called, Gauss. Adverse biological effects have been shown at 2.5 mG. That is why the recommended levels for constant exposure should be 1.0 mG or less. This is about the amount you would be exposed to if you were sleeping next to your electrical alarm clock. You can image the dose you are receiving when sitting in front of the computer under fluorescent lights chatting on the cell phone.

There are several ways to combat EMFs. Applying all of the health-building principles in this book will strengthen your immune system thereby making you more resilient. However, some people are so sensitive that they need some outside support. For these patients I check their need for an anti-EMF devise sometimes called a QLink or "Quantum Link."

What is a QLink?

According to the manufacturer, the technology that makes QLinks work is called "Sympathetic Resonance Technology". The QLink works according to the principle of resonance. Resonance is the phenomenon where one object in oscillation is able to cause a second object to oscillate at the same frequency. If both objects were already in oscillation, the stronger would eventually influence the weaker until the two were in harmony. Resonance also produces an amplification of the original frequency making its effect even greater. That is why the QLink is able to produce a therapeutic effect.

I remember how my old car would start to shake at a certain speed. The oscillation created from the tires rotating on the road surface would cause resonance with the loose parts on the car, nearly shaking it apart. Other examples would include: the plucking of a single guitar string that then caused the oscillations of the others; two tuning forks in close proximity where one is tapped causing the oscillation of the other; or an opera singer holding a note until a champagne glass shattered.

Studies from the Institutes of Heart Math have shown that your immune system is strengthened when you are engaged in joyful (positive) states of mind. Emotions are contagious. Think of how you feel when someone who is happy and vibrant comes into the room and engages you in conversation. Then think of how you feel when someone down and depressed comes in the room and begins to tell you all of their problems. The former will enhance your mood, while the latter may bring you down. This is a form of energetic resonance between people. The QLink is designed to amplify your mental, emotional and physical energy states, just like the happy person. The QLink is calibrated to only resonate with positive healthy energy states, which when amplified, produce a therapeutic effect.

What's inside the QLink Pendant?

The SRT Resonator™ inside your QLink Pendant is made up of three hardware components:

- The resonating cell. The resonating cell is the size of a watch battery and is made of a unique combination of 99.999% pure crystalline elements. It works as an oscillator to conduct subtle positive energies.
- The tuning board. The tuning board reinforces the resonating cell to function in a specific spectrum or energy range. It harmonizes and protects the functioning of the resonating cell.
- The amplifying coil. The amplifying coil is 75 feet of copper wire wound into approximately one inch in diameter. It shapes and strengthens the size of the energy field that is conducted.

Research on subtle energies and their effects on biological systems continue at universities throughout the world. For example the cytoplasmic granule flow within plants is greatly disrupted in the presence of artificial light. There are many other similar examples. Although the effects are sometimes seen, they are still not fully understood. I therefore use applied kinesiology as a verification tool if I believe a patient is sensitive to electromagnetic fields. Here is what I do:

1. With the patient standing I find a strong arm muscle (usually a shoulder muscle works fine).
2. I then have them touch a working light switch and retest the muscle.
3. If they stay strong, I introduce them to a stronger electromagnetic field. While the patient holds a hair dryer or other electrical devise that is *turned on,* I test to see if the strong muscle weakens.
4. If the muscle stays strong in both cases, there is a good chance that the patient is not sensitive to electromagnetic fields.
5. If the muscle went weak on either case I then retest them, this time while they are wearing the QLink. In most cases the QLink will negate the original weakness caused by the electromagnetic field.

Patients who do require a QLink often report that their energy is increased, their mind is less "fuzzy" and their sleep is deeper with fewer interruptions.

LABORATORY EXAMINATIONS

It is common for people to describe significant symptoms to their doctor only to then be dismissed because nothing was detected on one or more diagnostic tests: X-ray, MRI, blood samples, throat cultures and many more. The reason is that these tests are designed to detect a disease. However, symptoms are often present without a disease. The problem is functional not pathological. *A functional illness can be defined as a disruption in any of the body's systems without the presence of a disease.* In other words, the body, for whatever reason, is not functioning to its fullest potential. With a functional illness, a patient will have symptoms (sometimes debilitating ones) but their life is not in danger. The illness is a signal by the body that something is wrong.

Although the testing done through applied kinesiology is extremely helpful in the discovery of underlying functional problems, it is not perfect. I therefore occasionally rely on the help of certain laboratory tests. The ones I use are designed to detect imbalances in body chemistry that are present in both known disease and functional illness. They evaluate five different areas: the endocrine, immune, gastrointestinal, and metabolic systems as well as a comprehensive test for nutritional deficiencies. To complete these tests, usually a sample of saliva, blood, stool or urine is required.

To give you an idea of how these tests work, I will describe one that most people need: *The Adrenal Stress Index.*

The Adrenal Glands

Remember from the Philosophy chapter how accumulated stress takes its toll on all of our tissues and eventually leads to illness of all types. The adrenal glands (one on top of each kidney) have a special role to play when it comes to stress. They are the tissues that, if evaluated properly, will tell us just how bad the accumulated stressors are. They are also the tissues that, if treated properly, will help us overcome present illness and future stress. These glands are extremely important. I often tell patients that if they neglect to care for the adrenal glands, they should not expect to fully recover from their illness or injury and should not be surprised if they have other mysterious problems or conditions in the future.

Why Are The Adrenal Glands So Important?
The adrenal glands are your stress fighters. No matter what the stress, they respond with various types and amounts of hormones. These hormones assist the tissues under stress so that they may continue to perform. The adrenal glands make three categories of hormones:

- Mineralcorticoids (Aldosterone)
- Sex Hormones (Estrogen, Testosterone)
- Glucocorticoids (Cortisol)

When the adrenal glands are functioning properly they provide many benefits such as:

- Moderate the stress response
- Regulate mood
- Aid in blood sugar utilization
- Support the reproductive system
- Strengthen the musculoskeletal system
- Strengthen the immune system
- Promote regular sleep cycles

Adrenal Fatigue
Under longstanding or severe stress the adrenals begin to fatigue. Dr. Hans Selye studied the process of adrenal fatigue and called it the *General Adaptive Syndrome*. A quick look at the chart below demonstrates how important it is to have healthy adrenal glands.

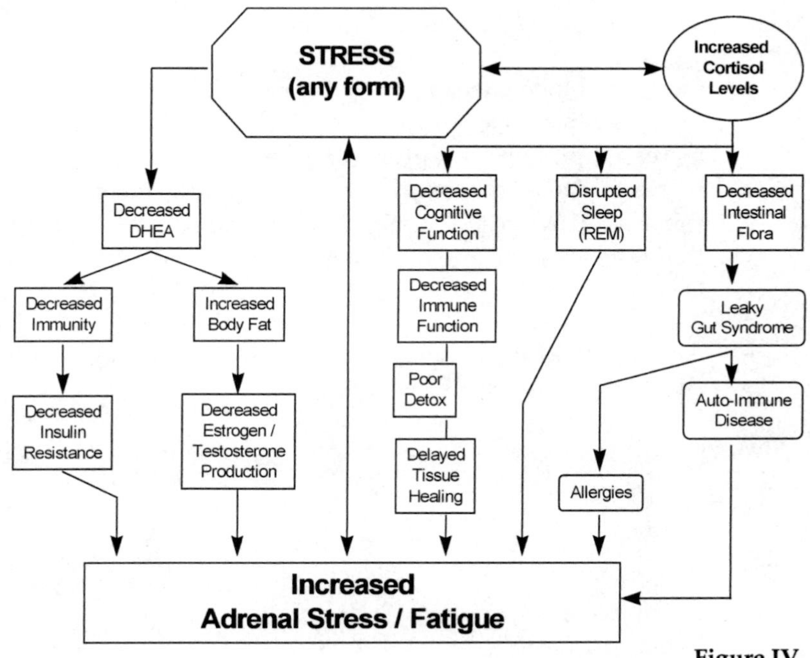

Figure IV

DHEA

You can see from the left side of the chart that the hormone DHEA is very important. This is one of the substances that may need to be given as a supplement when attempting to repair the adrenal glands. Like most hormones however, it should not be given for long periods of time, because the adrenal glands may stop producing it all together. Instead, like priming a pump, DHEA is given in small doses and for short periods. When done this way, the adrenals receive some rest and future DHEA production is encouraged.

Cortisol

Cortisol is the hormone we need to concern ourselves with most. If we can control the levels of this hormone we can correct adrenal function and improve health. Cortisol is a regulator and a balancer. Once in the blood stream, cortisol may prevent or encourage the release of hormones from other tissues. This is what it is supposed to do, but stress is not supposed to last indefinitely like it does for many people in this country. When this is the case, cortisol remains in the blood stream at high levels for a long, long time, resulting in some familiar conditions:

- Increased blood sugar (hypoglycemia).
- Increased insulin levels (diabetes).
- Increased protein absorption (muscle atrophy).
- Increased metabolic toxins like lactic acid (fibromyalgia).
- Decreased thyroid hormones (hypothyroidism).
- Decreased bone formation (osteoporosis).
- Delayed tissue healing.
- Loss of sleep (insomnia).
- Abnormal blood pressure regulation (hypertension).
- Fat production in the face and trunk.

Other specific problems that result from adrenal gland fatigue include:

- Fat storage
- Fatigue
- Dizziness upon standing
- Eyes sensitive to light
- Asthma
- Diminished libido
- Physical training burnout
- Inability to fully recover from illness or injury
- Acute pains for no apparent reason

The Adrenal Stress Index

One of the easiest ways to evaluate adrenal gland function is with a simple saliva test. Salivary testing is better than blood testing for two reasons. First of all, you don't have to draw blood, and second, the active adrenal hormones (the ones that are working) are all found in saliva. This test provides a great deal of important information and is inexpensive as far as laboratory tests go (around $109.00). I suggest that this test be taken by everyone interested in assessing overall health.

Taking the Test

A small kit contains four pieces of cotton, each inside a plastic tube. The tubes are clearly marked with the time of day for collection. The patient simply places the cotton under his tongue for 30-60 seconds until it is fully saturated. Then return the cotton back into the plastic tube and refrigerate. Repeat this process three more times throughout the day at the times indicated. When you are finished, place all four specimens back into the kit, attach the appropriate postage and mail it away. Within two weeks a report will be sent to the doctor for evaluation.

Treating the Adrenal Glands

Specific treatment for the adrenal glands often depends upon the results of the ASI test. Below is a sample graph from a returned ASI test.

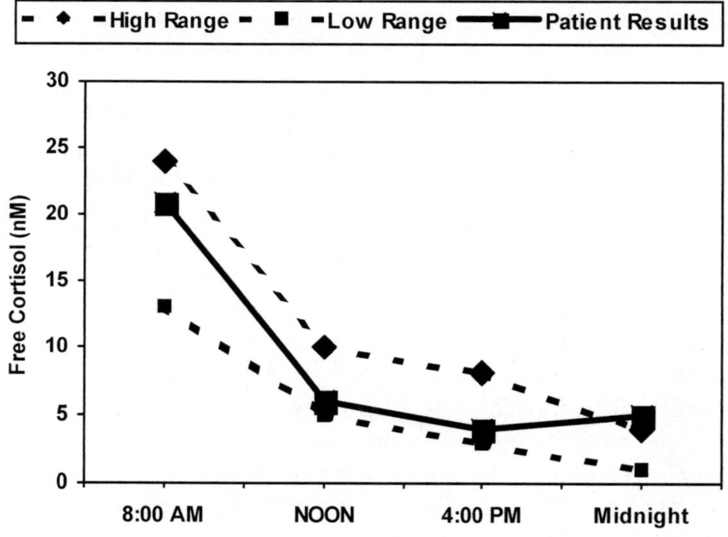

Figure V

You will notice from the above profile that the cortisol level at midnight is elevated, while all other levels are within the acceptable range. This usually means disrupted sleep, and sometimes depression. The goal in this case would be to lower the midnight levels only.

Correcting with Supplements

Phosphorylated serine has become a recent favorite of mine. This substance has the ability to either raise or lower cortisol levels. Many vitamins, including B vitamins contribute to the health of the adrenal glands as well. In fact, when stress is high, a large number of B vitamins are necessary in order to replenish the adrenal gland's nutrient pool. I also mentioned DHEA earlier. In more severe cases, adrenal hormones must sometimes be supplemented. Hormones themselves are complex chemicals made up of many other nutritional components found in the diet and in certain nutritional supplements. Diet, however, is not enough.

When the adrenal glands finally reach a depleted state and are thus fatigued, they have exhausted their reserves. Supplying an average amount of nutrients, like those found in a multiple vitamin, will simply not do. The nutrient imbalance must be treated with an imbalance to correct the disproportion. This means supplementing with a high level of proper nutrients - those that refill the nutrient pool. The adrenal glands will only improve when given the correct supplements in their correct amounts.

The other factor to consider with adrenal gland fatigue is "why." Why is this person experiencing elevated cortisol levels at midnight? What is the cause? Unfortunately, finding out the answer to that question is not so easy since any prolonged stress is a suspect. It is often the case that adrenal fatigue is the result of a combination of several stressors. In the case above, a detailed history revealed emotional, work-related and family stress. These are common. Other major stressors include: poor diet, over training, dependence upon chemical stimulants like coffee and soda, not enough sleep, and physical trauma.

The Whole Person

Whatever the causes, as many as possible must be addressed. If it is not possible to remove or correct all of the causes at one time, then patients must remain on cortisol-regulating and other adrenal supporting supplements until their circumstances change. The good news is that most patients experience high levels of improvement regardless, because enough stress is removed by fixing what can be fixed. Let me illustrate.

The adrenal glands are like a pump that uses water to put out a fire. Stress is the fuel with which the fire burns. Simply put, a fire can be extinguished with lots of water, or a fire can die out by removing the fuel. By supporting the adrenal glands with specific supplements, you in essence provide more water. By reducing stress through diet, exercise, and detoxification you take away the fire's fuel. Doing both at the same time is a sure way to fix the trouble.

The example above is typical of the kind of findings you can expect from a functional diagnostic test. This information would not have been found in a standard blood test and so, chances are the problem would have gone untreated for many years until something worse developed.

COMMON CHRONIC CONDITIONS

SECTION II

CHRONIC ILLNESS PROTOCOL

In this second section I will describe some of the common chronic conditions I treat every week in the office. I call them chronic because they have been part of a patient's life for six months or more. In most cases, by the time the patient reaches my office, they have been dealing with one or more chronic issues for many years. When treating any chronic illness I employ a whole-person approach. Remember from the chapter on Philosophy, that I strongly believe every part of the body is to some degree influenced by all the other parts. This idea can be clearly demonstrated when attempting to correct a chronic illness. In order for healing to take place, chronic illnesses require that all of the body's systems (structural, chemical, emotional) be addressed; often at the same time. This means that I will try to use as many stress-reducing tools as I can on each visit with the patient. The ones I frequently use are listed throughout Section I. However, the order in which these techniques are used can be just as important as the techniques themselves. It is my strong suggestion that even if the topic does not relate to your own health, you read all of SECTION III: *COMMON CHRONIC CONDITIONS*. This will allow you to gain a deeper understanding of the complexity of the human body and what it takes to correct dysfunction.

Eight Steps to Correct Chronic Illness
Below are the common steps I take to examine and treat a patient with a chronic illness. In a non-chronic illness, all eight steps may not be required.

1. **Check for subclinical infections** – A subclinical infection cannot be found on a blood test. Discovery often requires less orthodox techniques. Applied kinesiology is my tool of choice. Almost every person has some form of

subclinical infection. The highest percentage of those will be fungal. Elimination of these organisms is critical. For more information on the detrimental effects of microorganisms see: *COMMON CHRONIC CONDITIONS: Candida.*

a. Fungus

b. Virus

c. Bacteria

d. Parasite

2. **Check for food allergies** – It has been estimated that up to 80% of headaches are caused by some form of food allergy. When the immune system is suppressed from poor lifestyle choices, food allergies often result. For more information see: *COMMON CHRONIC CONDITIONS: Allergies.*

3. **Check for metal body burdens** – Heavy metal poisoning is becoming more of a problem than most realize. Symptoms can include everything from loss of memory to bipolar disorder. The removal of heavy metals from the body can be multifaceted. It is not unusual for symptoms to change or even temporarily get worse. The patient should be advised that removing heavy metals is a process that requires consistent treatment over the course of many months.

4. **Nutritional corrections** – Without proper rebalancing of deficient nutrients the body simply will not be able to function at a high level. Proper nutrition through diet and supplementation is critical. For more information see: *NUTRITIONAL THERAPIES: Supplementation.*

   a. Supply deficient nutrients

   b. Supply therapeutic nutrients – These are specific nutrients that benefit a given condition (i.e. L-glutamine and slippery elm bark for cases of intestinal inflammation).

5. **Desensitization** – This is the process where I use hands-on techniques to lower the body's response to a food (allergy) or an organism (infection). This step is done on all

chronically ill patients. If not performed 30% or more would not fully recover. For more information see: *COMMON CHRONIC CONDITIONS: Allergies.*

   a. Microorganisms

   b. Foods

   c. Chemicals

6. **Structural corrections** – Correcting structure even in cases where it seems unnecessary such as with allergies or digestive problems is often times essential. Nerves and muscles all have direct relationships with organs. Fixing unbalanced structure takes tremendous stress off the body as a whole making recovery quicker and more likely.

   a. Cranial & spinal adjustments – see: *STRUCTURAL THERAPIES*

   b. Reflex work – see: *APPLIED KINESIOLOGY*

7. **Emotional corrections**

   a. N.E.T.

8. **Lifestyle modifications** – These are critical in the initial recovery and for continued health once treatment has stopped. For more information see: *SECTION III: AT HOME.*
   a. Diet
   b. Exercise
   c. Stress reduction

Healthy Gut, Healthy You

The purpose of the gastro-intestinal tract, or gut, is multifold. Basically, it digests foods, absorbs nutrients into the blood stream, aids in detoxification, supports the immune system and eliminates waste. It is said frequently in the complimentary medicine community, "If you fix the gut, you fix the patient." That is because with almost every chronic illness some form of gut imbalance can be found. When I say gut, I mean the gastro-intestinal tract - the long continuous tube from your mouth to your anus. The gut is heavily protected by the immune system since what goes in may be harmful. In fact, 70% of the immune system is located within the linings of the gut. This, like all others in the body, is an appropriate design since food has great potential for contamination by organisms. Also, bad foods require an immediate immune system response so that the body may be cleansed.

When treating the gut, I primarily focus on the stomach, small intestine and large intestine. These areas have the greatest potential for immune suppression through a disruption in the normal intestinal balance, a condition known as *dysbiosis.*

There are over 500 types of organisms that reside throughout our intestines. They do us a great service when the relationship between them is good. Otherwise, a disrupted balance can lead to gas, bloating, constipation, diarrhea, immune suppression, inflammation and more. Correcting an upset gut is so important that of the steps listed above to correct chronic illness, the first five are related to intestinal repair. One of the most harmful disruptions of the intestinal system is an inflammatory condition known as Leaky Gut Syndrome.

Leaky Gut Syndrome

The lining of the gut is designed to only absorb nutrients from completely digested foods. However, when the lining of the gut is irritated through bad food, nutritional deficiencies, imbalances among the normal microorganisms (flora) or food allergies, the gut can become leaky. This means that undigested food particles can pass directly into the blood stream. This infiltration creates inflammation and an immediate immune (allergic) response. Auto-immune diseases such as Lupus Erythematosis, Multiple Sclerosis, Irritable Bowel Disease and Rheumatoid Arthritis, are examples of the immune system attacking the body's own healthy tissue. It is the opinion of many in the complimentary medicine world that auto-immune diseases are the result of many factors, one of which is a continuously active immune system. When the immune system has been overly active for a prolonged period of time it will eventually lose discernment – not recognizing the natural from the foreign.

The results of leaky gut are staggering.

- Chemical sensitivities.

- An overburdened and congested liver.
- Decreased IgA (immunoglobulin A) – a powerful part of our natural defenses. When decreased the body is not able to ward off protozoa, bacteria, viruses and yeast like candida.
- Intestinal inflammation – When present, bacteria and yeast are able to translocate. This means that they are able to pass from the gut lumen or cavity, into the bloodstream and set up an infection elsewhere in the body.
- Formation of antibodies – This is when allergies are established to certain foods. If not corrected, autoimmune diseases may result.

Here are some of the specific agents responsible for the creation of Leaky Gut Syndrome:

- Antibiotics lead to the overgrowth of abnormal flora in the gastrointestinal tract (bacteria, parasites, candida, fungi)
- Alcohol and caffeine (strong gut irritants)
- Foods and beverages contaminated by parasites like giardia lamblia, cryptosporidium, blastocystis hominis and others.
- Foods and beverages contaminated by bacteria like helicobacter pylori, klebsiella, citrobacter, pseudomonas and others
- Chemicals in fermented and processed food (dyes, preservatives, peroxidized fats)
- Enzyme deficiencies (e.g. celiac disease, lactase deficiency causing lactose intolerance)
- NSAIDS (non-steroidal anti-inflammatory drugs) like ibuprofen.
- Prescription corticosteroids (e.g. prednisone & hydrocortisone.)
- Diet high in refined carbohydrates (e.g. candy bars, cookies, cake, soft drinks, white bread)

- Prescription hormones like birth control pills and estrogen replacements.
- Mold and fungal mycotoxins (waste products) in stored grains, fruit and refined carbohydrates.

Leaky Gut Syndrome not only results in the development of food allergies, but it also allows the bloodstream to be invaded by bacteria, fungi and parasites that, in the healthy state, would not penetrate the protective barrier of the gut. These microbes and their toxins, if present in large enough amounts, can overwhelm the liver's ability to detoxify the blood. This results in symptoms such as confusion, memory loss, brain fog or facial swelling. Also, chemical sensitivities to cigarette smoke, gas fumes, perfumes and others, may begin to develop.

Leaky Gut Syndrome also creates a long list of mineral deficiencies. Even if the mineral levels are high in the diet they may not be getting to their target tissues because of inflammatory damage to carrier proteins. For example, a magnesium deficiency (low red blood cell magnesium) is a common finding in conditions like fibromyalgia (another common chronic condition, specifically of the muscles) despite a high magnesium intake through the diet or supplementation. Zinc, copper, calcium, boron, silicon and manganese are other common mineral deficiencies associated with Leaky Gut Syndrome.

The Up's and Down's of Chronic Illness

Correcting chronic illness is a process. Sometimes fantastic results are seen in the first few weeks. Other times the changes are slow and steady. It is also likely that there will be peaks and valleys as the patient learns to cope with their new lifestyle. For instance, if food allergies are part of the patient's condition, then an avoidance of the food becomes necessary for a period of time – and on rare occasions, indefinitely. If they eat the food in the future, they may begin to experience detrimental symptoms of some kind. This is a gentle reminder that this particular food is detrimental. Patients should see this response as a blessing and heed the warning of their body.

Inertia is the law that says that an object in motion tends to stay in motion unless acted upon by an opposing force. Likewise, an object at rest tends to stay at rest unless acted upon by an opposing force. The same applies to the chronically ill person. Remember that a chronic illness by definition has been a part of a patient's life for a long time. Poor lifestyle choices made over a lifetime have only permitted the body to move in one direction; an unhealthy direction. The result is both a metabolic and physiologic compensation. Symptoms such as high blood pressure, fatigue, joint pain, weight gain, anxiety, confusion and so on, are all examples. Continual compensation for bad choices without rest or replenishment is a significant stress that will eventually lead to a known condition or disease. The only way to restore health is to act in the body's best interest by applying a force in the opposite direction. This process will require work. And work, as we all know, is often times unpleasant.

There will be signs that the body is resisting change. From headaches to fatigue, any number of symptoms are possible. This makes sense given that the habits of the body have been firmly ingrained through years of bad choices. Some call these episodes a healing crisis; I simply call them *recovery symptoms.* The good news is that with our treatment programs most people experience very few if any recovery symptoms. For those who do, the highs are often much higher than the lows are low.

To give you a sense of the regularity with which I apply a whole person approach and just what kind of treatments I employ with chronic conditions, I created the table below. The number 1 means that the procedure is rarely required, while a 5 means that the procedure is always required.

Common Chronic Conditions	Desensitization	Diet Changes	Emotional Stress Reduction	Exercise Program	Specific Supplementation	Hands-on Therapies
Allergies	5	5	3	2	5	4
Candida	5	5	5	5	5	5
Depression	2	4	5	4	4	5
High Cholesterol	1	5	4	4	5	4
Heavy Metal Toxicity	5	3	3	3	5	5
Hormone Balancing	2	4	4	3	5	4
Hypoglycemia	1	5	2	3	5	4
Menopause Symptoms	1	4	3	3	4	2
Osteoporosis	1	3	2	5	5	5
Pain	2	3	2	3	3	5
PMS	2	4	4	4	5	4
Stress	2	4	5	3	5	4
Weight Loss	4	5	3	5	4	4

Figure VI

ALLERGIES

When most people hear the word allergies, thoughts of itchy watery eyes, sneezing and congested sinuses come to mind. What many do not know is that you may have allergies and never experience any typical allergic symptoms. In fact, allergies can be the cause of a whole range of seemingly unrelated health conditions including fatigue, headaches and chronic muscle pain.

What are allergies?

An allergic reaction is the result of our body's own immune system releasing certain defender cells (immunoglobulins) in response to a substance called an allergen. Allergens can be almost anything including: foods, dust, molds, pollens, chemicals, or even electromagnetic radiation. For the allergic person, even brief contact with an allergen can produce a severe immune system response.

In order to be properly classified as an allergy, one of two types of immunoglobulins, called IgE or IgG, must be present in a blood sample. However, many suffer from the identical symptoms but do not have a measurable level of IgE or IgG in their blood. Instead, these people have what are labeled food or environmental "sensitivities." Sensitivities and allergies are both treated successfully in our office by the same method.

Where Do Allergies Come From?

Remember from the previous chapter that a healthy gut usually means a healthy person and vice versa. Most allergies are in some way related to poor digestion or leaky gut syndrome which allows undigested food particles to enter the blood stream. The immune system immediately recognizes these particles as intruders and attacks by releasing histamine and other chemicals. It is this release that produces the familiar allergic symptoms (itchy eyes, runny nose, sneezing etc.).

Other allergies not directly related to excess gut permeability (i.e. pollen, dust or pet dander) are often the result of an immune system imbalance. The imbalance may be described as over-active (hyper) from either extended exposure to the substance or genetic reasons, or under-active (hypo) from excess stress. These imbalances may be corrected by fixing the gut.

Up to 70% of the immune system is located in the intestinal lining. It is our body's first line of defense. If the lining is compromised then so is the immune system, resulting in a potential allergy.

Once the gut lining has been compromised the chances for unfriendly organisms taking residence greatly increases. In fact, to correct most cases of leaky gut, the doctor must simultaneously treat to correct a foreign organism. Treatment is usually in the form of supplementation and "desensitization" to the organism itself (see below).

Restoring normal nerve communication
Allergies greatly upset the normal communication of the nervous and immune systems. Restoring communication is done through our low-force adjustive procedures, which are performed each visit as needed.

Re-establishing epithelial (gut) integrity
This is done through supplementation based on appropriate findings including the presence of organisms. It takes a minimum of three weeks for the gut lining to heal and longer if more than one of the following are present:

- Fungus
- Virus
- Parasite
- Bacteria
- Heavy Metals

Desensitization

Using Applied Kinesiology, the response of the body's structural, chemical and emotional systems are measured in both the absence and presence of an allergen. In the presence of an allergen the body "switches" to an adaptive/protective mode. When this event occurs, typical allergy symptoms are present along with other more subtle yet measurable signs identified with Applied Kinesiology testing. These include neurolymphatic, neurovascular, structural, and even emotional changes. Identifying and then reversing the subtle responses (desensitizing) is a key to the correction of allergies.

A patient can be desensitized to almost anything that produces a hyper immune response. This means that the immune system produces more allergen fighting chemicals than are required. Pets, chemicals, organisms (fungus, bacteria etc.), heavy metals and foods are the most commonly desensitized elements. In order for a desensitization to occur the patient must first be exposed to the substance. This initiates the immune response and produces a number of changes throughout the body such as subluxations, activation of reflex points, blockages within the energy system (meridians), muscle tension and more. Through processes not fully understood, correction of these changes, *in the presence of the allergen* will make the immune system less sensitive to the allergen.

Treatments take about fifteen to twenty minutes and are performed in-office. Following treatment the patient avoids the treated allergen for up to three weeks. This time period is critical to the success of the treatment. Without proper adherence to the prescribed protocol, long-term relief is not as likely. After the avoidance period, the patient may then eat or come in contact with the allergen and in most cases the allergy is completely eliminated.

Those who adhere to my treatment recommendations obtain excellent results. Our patients have reported consuming eggs and dairy products for the first time in years, the ability to sit in a room with cats, ridding themselves of allergy medications, sleeping through the night without the use of an inhaler, and reducing their overall pain.

What is the difference between this treatment and N.A.E.T?

Nambudripad Allergy Elimination Technique (N.A.E.T) was developed by a Dr. Nambudripad who specializes in acupuncture treatments for allergy desensitization. I do not use needles in this office. Instead I rely on subtle stimulation of acupressure points, neurolymphatic reflexes and other non-painful reflex points for the desensitization of an allergen. With N.A.E.T a patient must typically undergo a series of treatments for different groups of allergens. It is not uncommon to hear of a patient receiving thirty or forty treatments. Although this number of visits seems high, for the chronic allergy sufferer, relief is all that matters. Thankfully, our program significantly reduces the total number of visits. This is possible because our program addresses both the desensitization of the allergen itself and the correction of the imbalances that permitted the allergic reaction in the first place. N.A.E.T addresses only the former.

Conclusion

Allergies come in many shapes, sizes and varieties. In my opinion this technique is not just for eliminating allergies, but for strengthening the immune system. This leads to significantly improved health, and should be considered by all who desire to do just that.

STRESS

Stress is a natural part of life. Without stress we could not mature emotionally or physically. The dilemma occurs when the stresses of life overwhelm our abilities to cope – a common problem. In fact, stress produces adverse effects in 43% of all adults and is related in some way to 75% - 90% of all medical visits. Stress also contributes to chronic illnesses such as cardiovascular disease, diabetes, osteoporosis, gastrointestinal disorders, obesity, cancer, anxiety and depression. Often just the thought of a stressful event is enough to cause an increased heart rate, perspiration, or in severe cases, panic attacks.

When you say, "stress" most people think of situations that are extremely worrisome; a state where their minds are constantly occupied with a given situation. As the statistics just mentioned demonstrate, this kind of stress is detrimental to the health of the body. However, emotional stress is just the beginning. There is more than one kind of stress. Structural trauma and chemical deficiency or chemical toxicity, are also forms of stress with their own detrimental health effects.

Type of Stress	Description
Structural	These are stresses that affect primarily your muscles and joints. Examples include: overworking a muscle, wearing shoes with poor support, dental problems and any previous injuries.
Chemical	Whatever you eat, drink or breathe, is or can become a chemical stress. Also, an imbalance in your nutritional reserves is considered a chemical stress and permits the development of other chemical stresses.
Emotional	Tension, anxiety and depression are the primary examples of this stress. Emotional stress can affect mood, cognition, sensation, perception, learning, concept formation and decision making.

Figure VII

To the body, no matter what its origin, stress has the same effect on the tissues designed to combat it.

The Fight or Flight Reaction

When a stress is present, a chain reaction takes place within the endocrine (hormone producing) tissues. Beginning at the hypothalamus, a hormone called CRH (corticotropin-releasing hormone) is secreted that stimulates the next in command, the pituitary gland. The pituitary then secretes a hormone called ACTH (adrenocorticotropin hormone) that directly influences the adrenal glands.

The adrenal glands are your stress fighting glands. The hormones they make are designed to manage important functions within the body like blood sugar balance and to provide excitatory chemicals so that you can either, "fight or flee." Generally, these hormones once released, should perform their functions and then be broken down and eliminated by the body. However, prolonged stress keeps them at high levels in the blood stream; this will eventually lead to all sorts of problems. Here are the three stages of the stress response:

1. *Alarm* - This is the "fight or flee" stage. All of us go through this reaction everyday to varying degrees as we face life in the high-speed modern world.

2. *Adaptation* - Most patients who come into my office are in this stage. Their body has been dealing with one or more stresses for a prolonged period of time; so much so that they have now begun to experience nagging aches and pains, chronic allergies, fatigue or a host of other symptoms.

3. *Exhaustion* - If your body has been in the adaptation phase for too long it will lose its ability to cope. The adrenal glands will no longer be able to keep up and their levels of stress fighting hormones will drop.

The Adrenal Hormones
A pair of adrenal glands, one on top of each kidney, is responsible for the production of some important hormones. Keeping these hormones in proper balance is a key to the prevention of illness resulting from stress.

The glucocorticoids - These are produced by the adrenal glands in response to stressors such as emotional upheaval, exercise, surgery, illness or starvation. The most recognizable of the glucocorticoids is cortisol.

- Cortisol is one of the best hormones to evaluate when assessing the overall effect of stress. It has many excellent properties including being immune stimulating, anti-viral, anti-bacterial and anti-inflammatory. However, chronic elevated cortisol levels suppress the action of the immune system and predispose us to frequent infections. They will also lead to weight gain through fat storage and muscle tissue breakdown, a process called catabolism. Two diseases are associated specifically with cortisol. Cushing's Syndrome occurs when the body produces too much cortisol and Addison's Disease generally results from insufficient cortisol levels.

The catecholamines – These are any of several compounds occurring naturally in the body that serve as hormones or as neurotransmitters. The catecholamines include such compounds as epinephrine (adrenaline), norepinephrine, and dopamine. Epinephrine and norepinephrine are secreted by the inner part of the adrenal gland, called the medulla.

- Epinephrine is the primary hormone secreted when we are scared or nervous. It prepares the body for "fight or flee." It is a powerful hormone that is often used medically as a stimulant in cardiac arrest, as a vasoconstrictor (makes the blood vessels smaller) in shock, and as a bronchodilator (makes the lung vessels bigger) and antispasmodic in bronchial asthma.

Successful Stress Management

There are many successful approaches to lowering stress. By doing so you can expect to reduce your risk for chronic conditions, help control your weight, and improve your overall quality of life.

1. *Adrenal Stress Index-* Since the adrenal glands do much of the work required to properly manage stress, if your doctor wants to get an idea of how well they are doing, he can have you perform a simple test called an adrenal stress index. This is the saliva test I discuss in detail in Section I: Laboratory Examinations. This test does a great job of measuring all of the active levels of the hormone cortisol. If this hormone is out of range, it is likely that your adrenal glands have been working too hard.

2. *Stress List* - An effective way to reduce various stresses is by writing them down. On a piece of paper make three columns. In the first column record all of your structural stresses. In the second column record all of your chemical stresses. In the third column record all of your emotional or mental stresses. Once you have them recorded, try to prioritize them by putting a number or an asterisk next to the most significant ones. Finally, reduce the ones you can.

Structural	Chemical	Emotional
*Headaches	*Fast foods	Job
Sore feet	*Chewing gum	*Relationship w/ co-worker
R. Shoulder pain	*Sodas	Finances
Trouble sleeping	*Snacks	*Sick pet
Broken hand	Medications	

Figure VIII

Your stress list may look something like this. The chemical section is usually the easiest one to correct. Looking at the chart above, simply working on a better diet would help this person go a long way to reducing his overall stress. The other stresses will require different strategies.

3. *Warm baths with essential oils* – usually only 2 or three drops of a good essential oil are all that is required.
    - Lavender
    - Chamomile

4. *Relaxation techniques*
    - Stretching
    - Some forms of Yoga

5. *Diaphragmatic Breathing* – When you breathe deeply the expansion of your lungs stimulates the autonomic (unconscious) nervous system, specifically the parasympathetic part, which has a calming and relaxing effect on your body. This simple technique can be done anywhere or at anytime. Follow the steps below:

    1. Inhale through nose and exhale through mouth.

2. Breath deeply into your abdomen, feel it expand to a count of 4.

3. Pause for a count of 1.

4. Exhale slowly to a count of 4, allowing tension to release.

5. Repeat until you feel relaxed.

6. *Lifestyle Strategies*

    - Time management.
    - Set priorities.
    - Organize your day.
    - Delegate what you can.
    - Don't over schedule.
    - Let go of perfectionism.
    - Learn to say "no" when appropriate.

7. *Exercise (see: Section III: Exercise)*

    - Vital part of a stress management program.
    - Moderate amounts of low intensity exercise helps to balance cortisol.
    - Choose an activity that leaves you refreshed and energized.

8. *Get Adequate Rest/Sleep*

    - The repair process for cells and tissues occurs mostly during the night.
    - Sleep deprivation leads to accelerated aging.

9. *Diet and Nutrition*

    - Limit caffeine
    - Limit or avoid alcohol
    - Eat regular planned meals in a relaxed environment

- Key nutrients for stress include:
  - Vitamin C
    - Fruits and vegetables
  - Pantothenic Acid
    - Whole grains, legumes, cauliflower, broccoli, salmon, sweet potatoes, and tomatoes.
  - Vitamin B_6
    - Chicken, fish, whole grains, nuts and legumes.
  - Zinc
    - Protein rich foods, such as meat and seafood, eggs, and milk.
  - Magnesium
    - legumes, nuts, and whole grains, green vegetables

WOMEN'S HEALTH

Addressing female health issues usually requires the correction of hormonal imbalances. PMS, abnormal menstrual cycles, depression, endometriosis, uterine fibroids, and hot flashes are all consistent with hormonal irregularities. Elevated estrogen is the primary imbalance associated with many of the symptoms just listed, but not all. Elevated estrogen is a result of many factors including: glandular dysfunction, liver congestion, allergic reactions, fungal and other microbial infections, birth control pills, poor diet and environmental factors like pesticides and plastics.

HORMONE REPLACEMENT THERAPY (HRT)

In July of 2002, a large, in-progress study examining the effects of a widely used type of HRT medication called Prempro®, which combines the hormones estrogen and progestin, was halted by the National Institutes of Health (NIH).

The NIH took action because the hormones increased a woman's risk of breast cancer as well as heart disease, blood clots and stroke. The findings were published in *JAMA*, the Journal of the American Medical Association. A review of preliminary data found a 26 percent increase in breast cancer, a 29 percent increase in heart attacks and a 22 percent increase in total cardiovascular disease among women receiving the hormones compared with women who received a placebo.

Three months later a British HRT study was also stopped for essentially the same reasons. There had been hopes HRT could reduce the risk of coronary heart disease, but in fact the reverse appears to be true.

These results are not at all surprising to many operating in the realm of natural medicine. In fact, doctors have known for almost thirty years that estrogen replacement by itself increased the likelihood of some cancers. That is why in both of the studies above, artificial progesterone was also given along with estrogen.

Hormones are extremely complicated substances with powerful effects on their target tissues – the ones they were designed to influence. The practice of giving replacement hormones when they are shown to be low in the body is, on the surface, logically sound. However, digging a little deeper reveals a few potential problems. 1. This method does nothing to correct the reasons why the hormones were low in the first place, which may aggravate an already disharmonious relationship and 2. Since the process of hormonal production and release is dependent upon numerous positive and negative feedback steps, adding hormones into this delicate system is potentially problematic. The preliminary results of the two studies mentioned above bear this out. In my opinion, it is far wiser to do everything you can to reestablish the normal ebb and flow of hormone production and release before ever attempting HRT.

I do see a use for HRT in certain instances where a woman has undergone surgery for the removal of hormonal tissue such as a hysterectomy or thyroidectomy. Also, there are certain instances where an autoimmune or congenital disease has damaged hormonal tissues. In these cases, hormonal replacement is probably the best option. That being said, there is one practice that I find awfully disturbing.

Birth Control Pills

In my opinion hormone replacements in the form of birth control pills are one of the worst abuses of medical knowledge in recent history. I base this strong statement on many factors including my understanding of the human body, the dramatic increase in infertility rates, menstrual irregularities, and estrogen related cancer rates. For a medical doctor to prescribe birth control pills for a young girl with menstrual cramps and presume that he has acted in her best interest shows absolute ignorance of the sensitivity of endocrine balance. He has in fact set her on a course that is potentially life altering in the most negative sense. From a natural perspective, the belief that artificially controlling the most basic and fundamental cycle of womanhood and expecting that the consequences be mild, or that there be none at all, is in utter contrast to the fundamentals of logic and reason. One only needs to ask friends and neighbors if they know of any young women with ovarian cysts, fibroid tumors or who are having trouble getting pregnant. Or, on the other end of the spectrum, ask if they know any pre-menopausal women with breast or cervical cancer. Then find out if they were ever on the birth control pill or HRT. The answers might just surprise you.

There are two kinds of birth control pills. The first type keeps estrogen high so that follicle stimulating hormone and luteinizing hormone peaks don't happen (explained below). This prevents an egg from developing properly or prevents ovulation all together. The second type keeps progesterone high so the body thinks it's pregnant.

The Effects of Birth Control Pills

- They confuse the body's natural hormonal production which in the very least will eventually make menopause difficult.
- They can create fibroid tumors. Many times fibroid tumors spontaneously go away at menopause because of a drop in estrogen.
- They lower vitamin B6 levels which can lead to depression, food allergies, carpal tunnel syndrome, and sensitivities to electromagnetic fields.
- They can affect fertility.
- They can result in recurrent yeast infections.
- Other known problems include: excessive uterine bleeding, blood clots, hypertension, depression, vomiting, increased weight, kidney disease and ovarian atrophy.

I have spoken with women about the negative effects of birth control and described the list of potential symptoms above. They are shocked and often reply, "My doctor never told me that!" If a woman feels the need to use birth control pills for her own reasons, then she should at a minimum, be associated with a physician capable of monitoring their effects, who can support her therapeutically in every way, so that the potential detrimental consequences of artificial hormone ingestion are minimized.

The Female Sexual Cycle

A key to understanding many of the issues women experience is to understand the menstrual cycle. Although there is variation with the normal length of the cycle, certain trends are expected before, during and after ovulation. For instance, if a woman experiences unpleasant symptoms (cramps, headaches, bloating) prior to ovulation, it is likely that estrogen is involved since its levels drastically change at this time. Similarly, if symptoms are experienced just prior to menstrual bleeding, progesterone may be involved.

The female sexual cycle (menstrual cycle) should be a rhythmic cycle lasting between 20 and 45 days. Its purpose is to prepare a female's egg (ovum) for fertilization with a male's sperm and to prepare the uterus to receive and sustain the fertilized egg.

There are three different hierarchies of hormones to consider when discussing the female sexual cycle. The first comes from the hypothalamus and is called gonadotropin-releasing hormone (GnRH). Its job is to stimulate the anterior pituitary gland to secrete two important hormones, luteinizing hormone (LH) and follicle stimulating hormone (FSH). Finally, these two hormones act directly on the ovaries themselves which then secrete estrogen and progesterone.

Understanding these hormones further requires that we look at the female sexual cycle in detail. Most consider day one to be the first day of menstrual bleeding. This day is actually the end of some very important steps as seen below.

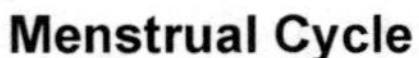

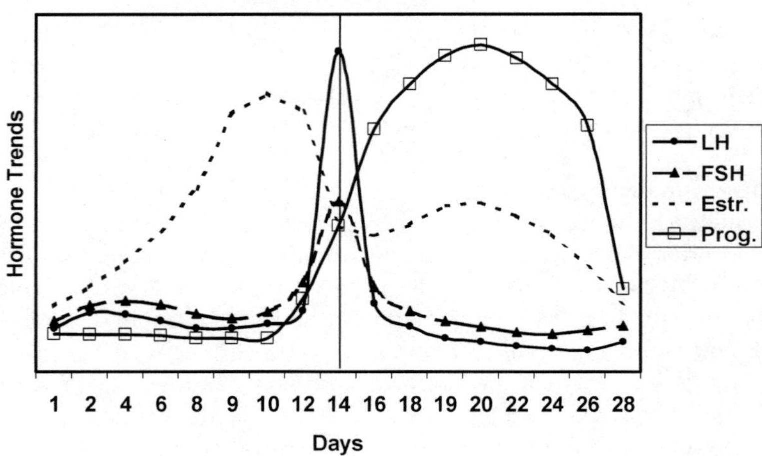

Figure IX

Synopsis

- Day 1: Shedding of uterine lining and gradual increases in estrogen from days 1 through 12.
- Day 12: Marked increase in FSH, drastic increase in LH, estrogen at its peak.
- Day 13: Dramatic drop in estrogen initiates ovulation.
- Day 14: Ovulation, FSH and LH at their peak, progesterone rising.
- Day 13: Surge in progesterone until day 23.
- Day 15: Drop in FSH and LH.
- Day 23: Progesterone at its peak.
- Day 24: Drop in progesterone until day 28.
- Day 28: lowest levels of progesterone initiates the shedding of the uterine lining (menstrual bleeding) on day 1.

Ovulation

For a woman with a 28 day cycle, ovulation occurs 14 days after the onset of menstruation. The first part of a woman's sexual cycle may vary from month to month by a few days, however, the last half of the cycle, from the time of ovulation to just before the start of menses, is usually a consistent 14 days.

A woman has about one million eggs when she is born. Once puberty begins, she releases six to twelve eggs each month. The eggs are contained within a follicle that grows under the influence of follicle stimulating hormone (FSH). One follicle will become dominant and cause the others to die off (become atretic). The sole remaining follicle will mature and eventually burst at the time of ovulation, releasing the egg within.

There are five characteristics of ovulation:

1. The rapid growth of the follicle by FSH.
2. Decreasing amounts of estrogen.
3. Increasing amounts of progesterone to promote pregnancy.
4. Release of the egg from the follicle.
5. A surge of LH to produce a corpus luteum.

Corpus Luteum

After ovulation the ovum is surrounded by a cloud of granulosa cells called a corona radiata. LH, which surges 6 to 10 fold two days before ovulation, changes the granulosa cells into lutein cells. Luteinizing hormone works primarily after ovulation to aid in implantation. The ovum and the lutein cells are called a corpus luteum. Over the next 6 to 12 days the corpus luteum will grow and secrete progesterone and some estrogen while awaiting fertilization. If none occurs, the estrogen secreted by the corpus luteum shuts off LH and FSH and the corpus luteum involutes or deteriorates.

Follicle Stimulating Hormone

FSH is designed to enlarge and grow the follicle. Its levels increase 2 to 3 fold at ovulation and drop within the next few days. With the absence of pregnancy hormones after ovulation FSH begins to rise again.

Estrogen

This is perhaps the most talked about hormone in the female cycle. It is responsible for the sexual characteristics of the female and causes the proliferation of many reproductive cells. Its job during the sexual cycle is to prepare the ovum for fertilization. Estrogen is high during the early part of the cycle and drops at ovulation. Too much estrogen is sometimes a cause for failed conception or can result in a failure to ovulate.

Progesterone "Pro Gestation"

Progesterone is the hormone most responsible for the healthy development of a baby. Many women who have trouble maintaining a pregnancy usually need some sort of progesterone supplementation. Its functions during the sexual cycle include: raising body temperature (incubation), preparing the uterus for pregnancy and the breasts for lactation, and inhibiting FSH and LH. If fertilization does not occur, progesterone drops, initiating menstrual bleeding due to the shedding of the uterine lining. If fertilization does occur, then a hormone called human chorionic gonadotropin (HCG) prevents progesterone from decreasing. HCG is the hormone that can be detected on a pregnancy test. If fertilization occurs, HCG will be present in the urine and blood stream around 1 week after ovulation.

The Causes of Hormonal Imbalances

Now that you have a basic understanding of the sequence of a normal hormonal cycle, here are some of the causes of hormonal imbalances. I have mentioned that hormone replacement is a bad idea because it does not address the underlying cause of why hormonal imbalances are present. Below is my list of ten causes, some of which doctors are completely unaware of, or have no idea how to treat.

1. *Poor diet* - A poor diet, those high in refined and processed foods, disrupts digestion which leads to inflammation of the linings of the small intestine. An irritated lining leads to poor absorption of nutrients (leaky gut syndrome). Poor absorption of nutrients leads to inadequate resources for the breakdown and processing of hormones and promotes the overgrowth of unwanted organisms such as candida.

2. *Plastic & pesticides* (xenoestrogens) – Plastics and pesticides that are absorbed into our bodies act like

estrogens. In lakes where large amounts of pesticides are dumped, fish become hermaphroditic, new born alligators are all female and the male alligators become feminized.

3. *Meats & milk* – This is another source of exogenous hormonal compounds with estrogen-like qualities. Last year 750,000 cows were injected with bovine growth hormone. They are also routinely injected with antibiotics and fed pesticide laden, genetically modified foods. As for milk, it is only as healthy as its source.

4. *Liver congestion* – The liver is the organ that does all of the breaking down of used hormones. If the liver is congested (full, fatigued, overworked) it does not have the resources to detoxify female hormones. As a result, the excess hormones continue to float freely in the blood stream, interacting with estrogen receptors on various tissues and creating a hormonal overload.

5. *Fungal infections* – This is an often overlooked cause of hormonal imbalances. It is very common for women to get yeast infections some time during the start of their cycle. Fungus (like Candida Albicans) feed on estrogen which increases the need for estrogen from the tissues. So, instead of a smooth increase and decrease of estrogen throughout the cycle, there is a series of peaks and valleys.

6. *Adrenal fatigue* – The adrenal glands are a secondary producer of estrogen. Messages from the pituitary gland force the adrenals to make more. However, since the adrenals are already tired, they do not meet demand and so the ovaries work overtime. Again, this means more peaks and valleys for estrogen.

7. *Allergies* – They increase inflammation in the tissues, which increases bloating and liver stress making the detoxification of hormones more difficult.

8. *Medications* – birth control pills and hormone replacement therapy (HRT). Although designed to correct imbalances, these often create their own.

9. *Nutritional Imbalances* – Proper quality and quantity of nutrients must be present in order for detoxification to take place effectively. Every illness has a nutritional

component. Without proper nutrition there will be much more wrong than just hormonal imbalances.

10. *Stress* – It is a powerful disrupter of adrenal gland function. The adrenal glands pay an important role in hormonal balance throughout the body. Please see: COMMON CHRONIC CONDITIONS: Stress.

The Results
Below I have briefly described the common conditions resulting from hormonal imbalances in women.

Menstrual Irregularities

PMS

Menopause

Depression

Osteoporosis

MENSTRUAL IRREGULARITIES

One of the most common gynecological problems is irregular menstrual cycles. Skipping periods, heavy bleeding, and spotting are all considered menstrual irregularities. When estrogen levels are high the lining of the uterus builds up in an exaggerated manner. This overproduction leads to a dramatic release of tissue at the time of menstruation and heavy bleeding results. Too much estrogen is usually associated with cramping, a shorter cycle and a longer period. Higher progesterone levels, on the other hand, usually mean light bleeding with little pain and a longer cycle.

When the overall level of estrogen is low, the uterine lining never properly forms and frequent release, or spotting, is likely. Too little estrogen results in vaginal dryness and in some women, hot flashes

PRE MENSTRUAL SYNDROME (PMS)

Researchers who study PMS estimate that as many as 40% of women suffer from this condition at some point in their lives. Bloating, acne, pain, emotional changes (moodiness, anger, depression), and fatigue are some of the common symptoms of PMS. Technically, in order to have PMS the symptoms must occur at the same time each month. For example, if a patient's symptoms were related to high progesterone they would be near the end of the cycle. Most PMS symptoms however, are related to excess estrogen and would therefore occur prior to menstrual bleeding.

Signs and Symptoms of Too Much Estrogen

- Breast swelling, fibrocystic breasts
- Water retention (edema)
- Premenstrual mood swings (depression)
- Loss of libido

- Uterine fibroids
- Heavy or irregular menses
- Craving for sweets
- Weight gain - fat deposition at the hips and thighs

MENOPAUSE

Menopause is officially the very last menstrual cycle. Most of the symptoms of menopause are actually pre-menopausal. They can occur either before or after the last cycle. In this case they would be called, peri-menopausal. Some symptoms include:

- *Menstrual irregularities* - longer frequency with shorter period
- *Hot flashes*
- *Vaginal dryness*
- *Numbness*
- *Insomnia*
- *Autonomic symptoms* – heart palpitations, pelvic pain, depression, mental instability, headaches, sweats, chills.

One of the main causes of menopausal symptoms is low estrogen. But with all of the environmental factors increasing estrogen in the female tissues, how can there ever be low estrogen? The answer is once again, the adrenal glands. Remember that the adrenal glands are secondary estrogen producers. When menopause hits, the ovaries greatly reduce their production of estrogen. If the adrenal glands are not healthy, they will not supply the missing amounts and low estrogen results even in the presence of high environmental estrogen.

Hot flashes, usually a symptom of low estrogen or low progesterone, are the most common complaint of menopausal women. Up to 80 percent of women experience them to some degree, with up to 40 percent suffering enough to seek medical attention. While some women never have a hot flash, most are inconvenienced by them for a year of two. For some women hot flashes may persist up to 5, even 10 years. I have found that balancing the body overall by correcting the causes of hormonal irregularities can have a dramatic effect on the frequency and intensity of hot flashes.

DEPRESSION

The cost of depression and other mental illnesses is between 30 - 300 billion dollars annually. Over 7 million women in the United States have clinical depression according to the National Mental Health Association. They are also twice as likely as men to be affected by depression.

Depression symptoms can include:

- A persistent sad, anxious, or "empty" mood.
- Sleeping too little, early morning awakening, or sleeping too much.
- Reduced appetite and/or weight loss, or increased appetite and weight gain.
- Restlessness or irritability.
- Persistent physical symptoms that don't respond to treatment.
- Thoughts of suicide or death.

Depression is a condition related to altered levels of a neurotransmitter called serotonin. Neurotransmitters are chemicals that stimulate specific receptors (neurons) in the brain producing a response. In the case of serotonin, when it stimulates its target receptors, a calming effect is produced which helps us to deal emotionally with the stresses of life.

In the person with depression, serotonin levels are low. This usually results from low levels of an amino acid called tryptophan. Tryptophan is converted into serotonin after several steps and in the presence of certain vitamins. Its effects are often experienced at Thanksgiving. Tryptophan is responsible for all of the sleepy relatives who have overindulged on turkey - a protein containing high amounts of tryptophan. In those with depression, there are three main reasons why this amino acid may be low.

1. *A low protein diet* - Since amino acids are the building blocks of protein, and tryptophan is an amino acid, if

there is not enough protein then tryptophan levels will be low.

2. *Poor protein breakdown.* All the protein in the world does you no good if your body lacks the ability to properly process it into its most basic parts - amino acids. This problem is often the result of low hydrochloric acid production in the stomach.
3. *Leaky gut syndrome* - If the protein is broken down properly in the stomach but the small intestine is inflamed and leaky, then absorption of the amino acids into the blood stream is compromised. Leaky gut is commonly associated with a food allergy or subclinical infection such as a yeast overgrowth.

When any of the three are present, supplementing with 5HTP, the substance that is converted into tryptophan, can be helpful until the above are corrected. Even if the levels of Tryptophan are sufficient there are two more reasons why serotonin levels may be low.

1. *Deficient vitamin cofactors* - Niacin, B6 and acetyl Co A are known to help in the production of serotonin. If these cofactors are low then the process will be inefficient at best and will likely result in low levels of serotonin.
2. *Competition with another hormone* - There is a fork in the road along the serotonin pathway. The body must choose between producing serotonin or melatonin - the hormone responsible for helping us fall asleep. Melatonin is generally produced under the influence of sunlight. Its production can be disturbed if you are constantly exposed to artificial lights, especially at night. Direct sunlight (no sunglasses) everyday is critical to proper pineal gland stimulation and melatonin production. Usually fifteen to thirty minutes is enough. If however, your job keeps you inside and you stay up late on the computer or go to sleep with the television on, chances are your melatonin production will be low. When this happens, the body must choose between the production of serotonin or melatonin. In most cases the body chooses sleep over mood. This is yet another reason why sleep is so important to our overall health.

The traditional correction of depression is through medications. There are two types of anti-depressant medications available on the market. The first is called an SSRI or selective serotonin reuptake inhibitor (brand names: Celexa, Luvox, Paxil, Prozac, Zoloft). This particular drug prevents neurons (nerve cells) from pulling in and recycling the serotonin that is floating in the space between neurons. This allows more serotonin to build up and continue stimulating its target receptors. The result is a more stable mood. The second type of medication is called an MAO inhibitor or monoamine oxydase inhibitor (brand names: Aurorex, Nardil, Parnate). Monoamine oxydase is an enzyme that breaks down serotonin so that its levels do not get too high. MAO's prevent this enzyme from doing its job. The result is therefore essentially the same effect as using an SSRI. More serotonin builds up between neurons, which equals an increase in activity. These drugs work very well. Unfortunately they have a number of side effects. MAO's for instance, have the inadvertent effect of increasing a chemical called tyramine. Monoamine oxydase enzyme usually breaks down this chemical. If an MAO-inhibitor is used, tyramine is not broken down. Elevated tyramine causes an increase in blood pressure, which could lead to stroke and heart attack. Because of this, people using MAO-inhibitors must avoid foods that are high in tyramine, such as alcohol, legumes (e.g., fava and soy beans), cheese, fish, ginseng, meat, sauerkraut, shrimp paste, soups, and yeast extracts.

Besides the side effects of anti-depressant medications, they do not address any of the reasons I listed above for low tryptophan and serotonin, and so the cause of depression remains. They also tinker with the body's natural hormone balance, which as you already know, I dislike very much.

There are many natural approaches to the correction of depression. Supplemental support with the proper cofactors, correcting food allergies and fungal infections, removing heavy metals like cadmium and mercury which are know to have mood altering effects, increasing sunlight and increasing exercise are all powerful tools to help restore normal brain chemistry. Often, combinations of these approaches are required.

OSTEOPOROSIS

Osteoporosis, the thinning of bone from decreased calcium and bone protein, is the most common bone disorder in America. More than 50% of healthy American women aged 30-40 are likely to develop vertebral fractures as they age due to osteoporosis. A woman may lose 30% to 50% of her cortical bone thickness over a lifetime. Some women lose bone much more rapidly around menopause. This phenomenon is believed to be related to a drop in estrogen levels. Preventive measures such as exercise, diet, and nutritional supplements are known to help prevent and partially reverse the effects of osteoporosis.

The body's priority is to keep *blood calcium* at its correct level.
It will therefore, sacrifice the available calcium in the bones in order to keep blood calcium levels adequate.

In order to ensure that you have plenty of calcium in your bones there are several things that have to happen.

- *Empty Stomach* - Calcium is best absorbed in an acid medium with a pH of 2 or less. This means that if you are using a calcium supplement you should take it on an empty stomach. Forget the idea of getting your calcium from an over-the-counter ant-acid, which is designed to neutralize acid and therefore make calcium absorption difficult. These companies have done a great job playing off of the calcium hype in the media by offering a calcium product to consumers that will do very little to meet their calcium needs.
- *Healthy Digestion* - Stress and a poor diet will lead to gut inflammation, making the absorption of calcium and all nutrients difficult.
- *Healthy Thyroid* - Calcitonin is a hormone produced in the thyroid gland. Its job it is to encourage calcium deposition in the bones by lowering it in the blood. If the thyroid is not working properly from a deficiency in the

amino acid tyrosine, for example, then calcitonin may be low.

- *Healthy Parathyroid* – A hormone called parathormone has the opposite function of calcitonin. Its job is to draw calcium out of the bones. It is made by the parathyroid glands. If this tissue is hyper, or working too much, it could lower bone calcium levels.
- *Proper Co-factors* - By itself calcium will not do anything to build bones. All of the other mineral and vitamins must be present in order to transport and bind calcium to the bone matrix. These include: boron, magnesium, copper, B vitamins, zinc, vanadium, chromium, vitamin D.
- *Sunlight* – This is the primary means of vitamin D production.
- *Weight Bearing Exercises* - Vigorous exercise stimulates the cells within the bones to produce more bone.
- *Avoid High Protein Diets* – These are good for short-term therapeutic results, but calcium is combined with protein metabolites as a flushing agent. Continued high protein diets will result in some calcium loss.
- *Avoid Soft Drinks* – Calcium is in a delicate balance with phosphorous. Sodas are very high in high phosphoric acid. When the blood levels of phosphorous are high, calcium (taken from the bones) is required as a neutralizing agent.
- *Avoid Caffeine* – yet another side effect to this more-popular-than-ever additive is that it lowers calcium in the bones.
- *Increase Seeds And Green Foods* – These are the foods of choice for increasing overall calcium levels.
- *Avoid Cow's Milk* – Yes cow's milk is high in calcium, so are the ant-acids I mentioned above. The problem is not the presence of calcium, it is the availability. If the calcium is in a form that is not easily absorbed, like cow's milk, then it will do you no good no matter how much you consume. Milk is also fraught with other problems as well. See: AT HOME: Diet.

BALANCING ESTROGEN

As you can tell by now, just like nearly ever other longstanding problem, balancing estrogen requires the combination of several therapies.

- *Balance Endocrine Glands* - The hierarchy:
    - Pineal gland
    - Hypothalamus
    - Pituitary
    - Adrenals
    - Thyroid

The above is accomplished with nutritional support, glandular products, natural progesterone (in the case of high estrogen) and stress reduction.

- *Nutritional Supplementations*
    - Vitamins: E, C, Alpha lipoic acid, N-acetylcysteine, B6, B12, Folate.
    - Minerals: Selenium, Calcium D-glucarate, Magnesium.
    - Herbs: milk thistle, dandelion, black cohosh, chasteberry, ginseng, dong quai, and licorice.
    - Oils: Fish, flax seed, black currant seed
    - Others: Indole-3-Carbinole (found in cruciferous vegetables.), curcumin.

- *Foods* - Phytoestrogens – These plant compounds have both estrogenic and anti-estrogenic effects. This means that if estrogen levels are low they work to bring them up. Likewise, if estrogen levels are high, they work to bring them down.
    - Isoflavones – Soy, legumes, alfalfa, clover, licorice root and kudzu root.

- Ligans – Increase SHBG (binds to hormones and reduces their effect) in the liver; inhibit aromatase activity (where your fat cells actually produce estrogen). Found in high fiber foods, whole grains, seed oils, legumes and vegetables.

- *Removing microbes* – Microorganisms often feed on estrogen which has the temporary effect of decreasing estrogen levels. The body responds by making more. See: COMMON CHRONIC CONDITIONS: Candida.
- *Eliminating allergies* – Allergies increase inflammation and water retention. The liver, besides processing excess hormones, has the additional responsibility to eliminate the additional inflammatory waste products. See: COMMON CHRONIC CONDITIONS: Allergies.
- *Diet Changes* - Reduce sugar, caffeine, alcohol, nicotine, chocolate, bad fats, salt, and hormone foods. See: AT HOME: Diet.
- *Vigorous exercise (40+ min 4x/week)*
- *Hands-On Therapies* – Applied Kinesiology

    1. See which hormones weaken strong indicator muscles. This response probably means that these hormones are too prevalent in the body and need to be reduced. - Determine which nutrients are needed to break them down.

    2. See which hormones strengthen weak indicator muscles. This response probably means that these hormones are low in the body and that increasing them will be therapeutic. - Use foods & nutrition to promote the increase of these hormones.

HYPOGLYCEMIA

Carbohydrates are one of three macronutrients. The other two are proteins and fats. They are called carbohydrates because they are made up primarily of carbon, hydrogen and oxygen. They include: sugars and starches like breads, pastas, grains, syrups, candies etc. When broken down, carbohydrates form simple sugars that the body uses for "quick" energy. Although necessary in a healthy diet, if eaten to often they can produce a detrimental state in the body called Carbohydrate Intolerance.

Carbohydrate Intolerance (CI) is defined as the inability to properly metabolize ingested carbohydrates. This common phenomenon is usually related to insensitivity to the hormone insulin and usually results in blood sugar problems like hypoglycemia. Here is a list of the ten most common complaints by people with CI:

- *Physical fatigue* - Whether you call it fatigue or exhaustion, the most common feature of CI is the feeling of tiredness.
- *Mental Fatigue* - Frequently manifested as an inability to concentrate. Loss of creativity, memory loss, failing grades, and "learning disabilities" are other symptoms. These symptoms usually occur immediately following a heavy meal.
- *Low blood sugar* - Brief periods of low blood sugar are normal throughout the day especially if meals are not eaten on a regular schedule. But prolonged hypoglycemia associated with the following symptoms is not normal:

agitated and moody, jittery, dizzy, and craving sweets or caffeine. These symptoms usually abate dramatically when food is eaten.

- *Intestinal bloating* - Most intestinal gas is produced from carbohydrates. The gas tends to build and is worse throughout the day (and night).
- *Sleepiness* - Many people with CI become sleepy immediately following a meal containing more than their limit of carbohydrates. These are usually pasta meals or protein meals with bread or baked potato and dessert.
- *Increased fat storage and weight* - Many people have too much stored body fat. In males, an increase in abdominal fat is the first sign of CI. In females it is more common in the upper body and face.
- *Increased triglycerides* - High triglycerides in the blood are frequently seen in overweight persons. But even non-overweight people may have fat in their arteries as a result of CI. These fats are a direct result of carbohydrates being converted by insulin into circulating triglycerides. Fasting levels of 100 triglycerides may be indicative of a problem and a level of 150 is indicative of an insulin problem.
- *Increased blood pressure* - Most people with hypertension produce too much insulin and are CI. A direct relationship exists between insulin levels and blood pressure. Sodium sensitivity is common for these people. When eaten, the sodium further raises the blood pressure and promotes water retention.
- *Depression* - Carbohydrates are a natural "downer." This is the result of increased serotonin production in the brain. Serotonin is a neurotransmitter which has an inhibitory (relaxing) effect on the nervous system. That is why hotels sometimes place a piece of candy on your pillow at night – it helps you sleep by increasing serotonin.
- *Difficulty breaking addictive habits* - CI is prevalent in persons suffering from alcohol, nicotine, caffeine, drug or other chemical addictions.

The people most vulnerable to CI are those under stress, athletes who over train, those taking estrogen, those with a family history of diabetes, heart disease or stroke, and people over the age of forty. Without proper treatment, CI can lead to greater insulin resistance and serious disease.

There are a number of things that are helpful for correcting hypoglycemia and CI. When aggressively undertaken, a patient can often expect noticeable benefits in only a few weeks.

- *Specific nutrient replacement* - Vanadium, chromium, lipoic acid and other are used to balance blood sugar.
- *Dietary modification* - A low carbohydrate diet is required. Meals usually need to be smaller and more frequent - approximately every two hours.
- *Exercise programs* - Building a fat-burning metabolism is a must. This requires that an aerobic exercise program be maintained for several months without doing any anaerobic exercise (see: SECTION III: Exercise)
- *Hands-on therapies* - Structural corrections of muscle and joint imbalances are a must. This rebalancing removes large amounts of stress allowing for greater function of the immune and nervous system.

CHOLESTEROL

What is it?

Cholesterol is a steroid normally found in every cell of our body and is essential to life. Cholesterol is part of the membrane of all cells, works to build and repair cells, and produces hormones such as estrogen and testosterone. Its main job however, is to be converted into cholic acid in the liver (up to 80% of all cholesterol becomes cholic acid). Cholic acid is combined with other substances in the liver to produce bile salts, which aid in the digestion and absorption of fat. The body produces about 70% to 80% of its own cholesterol. Only 20% to 30% of cholesterol comes from the diet.

Measuring the blood levels for cholesterol is part of a routine physical and is a very good idea. There are three things that need consideration when looking at your cholesterol results: high density lipoprotein (HDL), low density lipoprotein (LDL) and triglycerides. Doctors differ as to the meaning of these substances at various levels. Most traditionally trained doctors would agree that:

- Total cholesterol below 200 mg/dl. is good and anything over 240 mg/dl. indicates that you are at risk for developing coronary disease.
- LDL cholesterol should measure below 130 mg/dl.
- HDL cholesterol should range between 35 and 40 mg/dl.
- If the HDL cholesterol reaches 60 mg/dl. or higher, you have a reduced chance for a heart attack.

- Triglycerides should be less than 200 mg/dl.

Although these numbers are a good guideline there are a few exceptions that are worth noting. Many complimentary doctors who deal in the functional realm evaluate these numbers in the following way:

- Total cholesterol should range from 150 to 220 mg/dl.
- HDL (the "good" cholesterol) should be at least 25% of the total cholesterol.
- LDL should be less than 120 mg/dl.
- Triglycerides should be less than 50% of the total cholesterol.
-

Triglycerides are a particular form of fat that is transported through your blood to the tissue. The majority of your body's fat tissue is made up of triglycerides. However, high levels of triglyceride in the blood can be a risk for heart disease.
Serum triglycerides come from two sources. The first source is the foods that you eat. If you consume a meal containing a lot of fat, your intestine will package some of those fats and transport them to your liver. The second source is your liver. Once the fats are received by the liver, it then takes fatty acids released by your fat cells and bundles them up as triglycerides, which are then sent out to the rest of your body to use as fuel.

The triglyceride level, not cholesterol, is often the key to understanding if a patient is at greater risk for a heart attack. Here are two examples:

Patient A:	Total cholesterol:	280 (above normal)
	LDL:	175
	HDL:	70
	Triglycerides:	130
Patient B:	Total cholesterol:	180 (normal)
	LDL:	97
	HDL:	35
	Triglycerides:	185

Patient A, would be strongly considered for pharmaceutical intervention, but are they really in trouble? It is true that their total cholesterol is above the normal range but the HDL number is greater than 25% and the triglycerides are less than 50%. This patient is actually doing well.

Patient B, on the other hand, is within normal limits on all of their levels. However, their triglycerides are more than 50% of the total cholesterol, and their HDL is less than 25% of total cholesterol. Patient B is actually at greater risk for a heart attack even though they have measurements within the standard normal limits.

Why Cholesterol is High?

There are at least four understood reasons why the cholesterol level may be elevated: 1. Too much is being produced by the body; 2. Too much is being eaten in the diet; 3. Improper cholesterol breakdown by the body (nutritional deficiency); 4. Under (hypo) functioning of one or more hormone producing tissues (usually thyroid or pituitary).

Correcting High Cholesterol

The three major methods of cholesterol manipulation that I use are dietary measures to reduce total cholesterol intake, nutritional therapies to enhance cholesterol breakdown and exercise to improve one's overall physiology.

Dietary Measures

It has been believed for many years now that cholesterol in foods is bad and contributes to heart disease. In fact, the type of food ingested is more important than whether the food contains cholesterol. Saturated fat for instance, will increase the blood concentration of cholesterol by as much as 25%. This occurs when the fat is taken to the liver, broken down and then manufactured into cholesterol. When cholesterol is eaten in the diet, however, the formation of cholesterol is stopped in the liver. This is called a feedback loop, and it prevents the level of cholesterol in the blood from increasing much. Therefore, eating saturated fats can have a much greater effect on the total cholesterol than can eating cholesterol itself. This does not necessarily mean that eating saturated fat will lead to atherosclerosis and heart disease.

Fats

Because of their supposed connection with heart disease and high cholesterol, fats are definitely a four-letter word in our society. But are they really bad? Cultures around the world that have diets historically high in saturated fat DO NOT have heart disease like we do in America. In some cases, like the Eskimos of North America or the Masai tribes of Africa, heart disease is non-existent despite extremely high dietary levels of meat and saturated fat. The scientific evidence, honestly evaluated, does not support the assertion that "artery-clogging" saturated fats cause heart disease. In fact, most of the fat found in clogged arteries is poly<u>unsaturated</u>. These fats cause many health problems because they tend to become oxidized or rancid when exposed to heat through cooking. Excess polyunsaturated oils like corn, soy, safflower and canola oils, have been shown to cause several diseases including: heart disease, immune system dysfunction, organ damage, digestive disorders, depressed learning ability, impaired growth, and weight gain.

Here is a list of some of the benefits of fats:

- Make up 50% of the membrane around all cells.
- Assist calcium transport and absorption into our bones.
- Protect the liver.
- Protect against harmful microorganisms.
- Primary fuel source for the heart and other tissues.
- Enhance the immune system.
- Enhance the nervous system.

Fats are essential. Without them we could not survive. But they need to be present in the proper ratio and be of high quality. The popular notion that fats must be avoided at all costs is absurd and has led to increased consumption of two categories of unhealthy foods: fat free foods and foods with high amounts of sugar. These have more to do with disease, including high cholesterol, than fat ever did. A third category of foods that increase cholesterol may be the unhealthiest of all.

Synthetic Fats

All fats are not created equal. Man-made synthetic and processed fats interfere with cholesterol breakdown and should be avoided. The process of partial hydrogenation changes the shapes of natural fats and oils so that they interfere with, rather than promote, normal fat metabolism. These processed fats are in nearly everything we buy in the grocery store, from salad dressings to candy bars, and from chips to breads. Partially hydrogenated fats and oils block the normal conversion of cholesterol in the liver causing an elevation of cholesterol in the blood. Margarine, which is often touted for its lack of cholesterol, is produced from partially hydrogenated fats. One of the biggest cases of misinformation in recent history is the suggestion that eating margarine instead of butter will reduce cholesterol. It is true that butter contains cholesterol and that margarine does not. But butter also contains high levels of normal fat mobilizing nutrients, and hence is a whole food, designed to take care of its own fats if eaten in moderation. Margarine can actually increase cholesterol levels.

The same facts are true for eggs. Egg yolks are one of the highest sources of cholesterol. But they are also one of the highest sources of natural fat mobilizers. Eggs and butter are two examples of whole foods, which in some people are actually useful for lowering cholesterol and improving fat metabolism. They should be avoided by patients with severely elevated cholesterol such as those who have a family history of poor fat metabolism and breakdown. Margarine, on the other hand is a synthetic fat whose consumption interferes with cholesterol metabolism and many other body mechanisms. Like other partially hydrogenated fats, it should be avoided by everyone.

Which Diet is Right? - Blood Analysis

Generally speaking with regards to diet for a patient 20 pounds or more overweight:

- If the triglycerides are high and the cholesterol is normal the patient should use a *low carbohydrate diet* to restore proper levels (example: The Atkins' Diet).
- If the triglycerides are less than 50% and the total cholesterol is high the patient should use a *low meat, high*

fruit and vegetable diet to restore proper levels (example: The Fit for Life Diet).

Nutritional Measures

Nutritional factors that help to lower cholesterol include adequate (but not excessive) levels of vitamin A and C, specific B vitamins, especially niacinamide (B3). Magnesium, zinc, chromium, and trace elements can also increase the level of HDL. Also useful are fat/mobilizing substances including choline and betaine (remember that most cholesterol is broken down to cholic acid in the liver). I use Applied Kinesiology to determine exactly what nutrients your body requires to help with the breakdown of cholesterol.

The most important factors in lowering cholesterol are the ones that naturally help the body to break it down, such as normalizing bowel function and exercise.

Normalizing Bowel Function

Many people have imbalances between the friendly and unfriendly bacteria in their digestive systems. Unfriendly bacteria cause a negative feedback to the liver, which interferes with cholesterol breakdown, causing blood levels to rise. Eating refined sugars and starches contributes to this imbalance in the intestines. Avoid processed sugars and starches and replace them with natural forms of complex carbohydrates, which are roughage-containing foods such as whole grains, fruits, and vegetables. These will both improve the bowel function and lower cholesterol levels.

Exercise Measures

The proper type of exercise will also help lower bad cholesterol (LDL) while increasing good cholesterol (HDL). Aerobic exercise is not the same thing as "aerobics". Aerobic exercise means performing continuous exercise using the same muscles over and over *while keeping your heart rate below eighty percent of its maximum*. Aerobic exercise utilizes oxygen to burn fat, which is good for keeping cholesterol at its proper level. Most people doing "aerobics" are actually exercising anaerobically. This means they are burning glycogen (stored sugar) instead of fat for fuel. Anaerobic exercise burns sugar in the blood and muscles and promotes fat storage.

The best types of aerobic exercise involve the continuous use of the leg muscles such as walking or riding a bike (see: SECTION III: Exercise)..

Summary

- Eat good fats (see SECTION III: Diet)
- Avoid refined foods
- Avoid synthetic fats
- Supplement your diet with cholesterol lowering nutrients
- Have your thyroid checked
- Exercise

CANDIDA

For many years Candidiasis, the overgrowth of certain intestinal yeast called Candida Albicans, was not recognized as a serious health issue. Doctors would not consider Candida as a potential health risk, because it is found in the intestines of all people. Recently, things began to change. It is now recognized that Candida Albicans is causing health problems for over 30 million men and women every day. Candidiasis is a major contributing factor or cause of:

- Allergies
- Anemia
- Chronic Fatigue
- Immune weakness
- Systemic degeneration

The last two by themselves add up to over two-dozen known health problems with sixty or more symptoms. Because of its seriousness as an infection and its ever-growing prevalence, a few descriptions and explanations are necessary so that we may be more aware of this topic.

Etiology

Soon after birth, the microorganism Candida Albicans is normally found in the intestinal tract of healthy individuals. It co-exists with many other microorganisms in a "friendly" form. However, under certain conditions, Candida may be encouraged to change its structure to the "unfriendly" mycelial form. It is this second form that must be treated and eliminated. Mycelia are root-like structures that are able to penetrate into other tissues like the gastrointestinal wall. This penetration breaks down the protective barrier, allowing many foreign substances to enter and pollute the bloodstream. The results are usually allergic reactions, fatigue, immune system disorders and many other health problems.

Candida itself may also pass through the intestines and enter the bloodstream. Once there, it can have far-reaching effects on almost any other tissue. This is why, for women, vaginal yeast infections are often a recurrent problem. If the yeast in the vagina has arrived there because of a compromised intestine, locally treating the infection will not result in a cure.

A yeast cell produces over 75 known substances that are toxic to the human body and interfere with normal food absorption. Candidiasis can therefore be a dangerous condition for the elderly and those with longstanding illness.

The Major Predisposing Factors

Here are some factors that tend to cause Candida to change from the passive to the aggressive form:

- *Loss of Natural Control Mechanisms* - Wide-spectrum antibiotics destroy the good and healthful bacteria (probiotics), which control the candida population. For example, probiotics compete with Candida for space and nutrients in the intestinal tract. They also release acid, which makes the environment less favorable for candida growth and even feed off the candida directly. When antibiotics kill probiotics, candida proliferates and can change to its pathogenic mycelial form. Prolonged antibiotic use will often result in Candidiasis symptoms that may linger for a lifetime if left untreated.

- *A Weakened Defense* - A number of factors can compromise the effectiveness of the human immune system. Lowered immunity may result from prolonged illness, stress (all forms), pharmaceuticals, alcohol abuse, smoking, lack of exercise, lack of rest, and poor nutrition.

- *Females* - Females are somewhat more susceptible to Candidiasis than males for several reasons. First, hormonal levels in females fluctuate with regularity due to the menstrual cycle. High levels of hormones such as estrogen tend to impair immune system function and stimulate the growth of candida. Women may also take birth control pills. These synthetic hormones are just as bad as natural hormones and produce the same or worse effects. And finally, in the female system, it is easier for Candida to pass from the colon to the urinary and reproductive systems. Vaginal yeast infections are a common result.

- *Creating a Breeding Ground* - Because of highly refined foods such as flour and sugar, the once healthy large intestines of most Americans are now a breeding ground for Candida. American foods are highly processed, low in nutrients and low in fiber. They have a tendency to "cake" to the walls of the intestine where they putrefy, turn rancid and ferment. This is the perfect environment for Candida.

Getting started

I specialize in desensitization protocols for microorganisms, food allergies and chemical disturbances. Being desensitized to Candida is a major catalyst for recovery. By simply using diet alone you must be very strict. Popular books dealing with Candidiasis recommend diet changes that, if adhered to, may take six months to one year to reverse the effects of the infection. Yeast is one of the most aggressive microorganisms around. You cannot have a bad day dieting when you are trying to get rid of yeast. Thankfully, my protocol, which includes diet, lifestyle recommendations and hands-on treatment, usually takes less than six weeks.

Die-Off

When Candida organisms are killed, large amounts of toxic material is rapidly released. This is called a "die-off" or a Herxheimer reaction. Die-off can produce certain uncomfortable effects such as flu symptoms (stuffiness, headache, general aches, and diarrhea), skin rashes, vaginal irritation/discharge, or even something unusual like numbness in the legs or mental confusion. These symptoms, although unpleasant at the time, are very temporary. One way to fight against this phenomenon is to support the detoxifying tissues since they incur the greatest burden. This is done with nutritional supplements. Patients rarely complain of adverse reactions when the proper supplements are given.

Correcting Candidiasis

To correct Candidiasis quickly and in most cases, permanently, requires a four step process.

1. *Desensitization* – the process through which your body no longer reacts adversely to the presence of yeast and yeast byproducts.

2. *Diet modification* – to ensure that the yeast growing in the gut does not receive its desired food for reproduction. For my recommended diet, see: SECTION IV, Yeast Diet.

3. *Nutritional supplementation* – to ensure that the body chemistry is in balance and to kill overgrown yeast.

4. *Structural and/or emotional corrections* – to ensure that as much stress, in whatever form, is being reduced and eliminated, giving you a better chance at a full and complete recovery.

If all goes well, it is not uncommon for a patient to overcome Candidiasis within three to six weeks.

PAIN

It is common in our fast-paced, pill-popping society to expect a quick fix whenever a problem arises. This scenario is often unrealistic and in many cases is undesirable. That is because stopping pain may undermine what the body is doing or "saying."

Pain results from the stimulation of pain receptors (nociceptors) by noxious stimuli. Noxious stimuli are usually one of three things: a build-up of common inflammatory substances, the internal fluids of damaged cells, or toxic levels of waste products from normal cellular functions.

There are many reasons for pain. Here we have broken them down into structural, chemical and emotional.

Structural reasons for pain

Pain results when structures like bones, ligaments, muscles or other soft tissues are injured. Injuries can occur from a single traumatic incident or over time from overuse. Once injured, pieces of damaged tissue and cellular material are released into the bloodstream and produce the chemical response known as inflammation.

Chemical reasons for pain

These are by far the most complicated. Below is a list of seven causes of pain from chemicals:

- *Lactic acid and other metabolic by-products* – These are released during athletic performance or strenuous activity.

- *Electrolyte depletion* – Related to athletic performance or inadequate replacement from the diet or supplements.
- *Hormonal imbalances* – These are caused from stress, inadequate intake of required nutrients, surgical removal of hormone producing tissues (ex. hysterectomy), or resulting from a combination of any of the seven imbalances.
- *Free radical propagation* – Results from inadequate antioxidant intake, or prolonged exposure to noxious chemicals (ex. Bleach, certain beauty products, or unknown hazardous environmental agents).
- *Fatty Acid imbalance* - Eating hydrogenated or partially hydrogenated fats creates a vicious cycle of pain and promotes many other harmful processes. Most people need the addition of either omega 6 or omega 3 fats into their diets, usually not both. Omega 6 fats include: safflower, sunflower, peanut and black currant seed and corn oils. Omega 3 fats include: flax seed, cold water fish, EPA and olive oils. Over-the-counter pain medications (NSAIDS) and "good" fats work along the same chemical pathway to control inflammation. Therefore, you know you have an imbalance in essential fatty acids if taking NSAIDS reduces your pain.
- *Histamine reactions* - These occur in the presence of an allergen and usually mean a runny nose, itchy eyes, sneezing etc. Many histamine reactions are present without symptoms. They create inflammatory responses that produce pain.
- *Kinin Reactions* - This is another form of allergy. It is slower and tends to cause stuffiness instead of sniffling and sneezing.

Emotional reasons for pain

Pain is registered in the emotional centers of the brain. Because of this, the severity of pain can be greatly over-exaggerated or almost completely suppressed depending upon the mental make-up of the person. It should be stated however, that the presence of chemical or structural injury will greatly affect ones ability to control the perception of pain.

Hopefully, the information above helps you to understand that pain is multifactorial and therefore quite complicated. This is why I am convinced that the whole-person approach, using combinations of therapies to promote health, is not only the most effective, but the most prudent and the one that my patients deserve.

LOW BACK PAIN

Low Back Pain

Low back pain is as serious a problem as it is common. Low back pain is the second most common reason for physician visits among all Chronic Pain disorders. 60-80% of all people will have low back pain sometime in their lives. 15% of these will be disabled as a result. Concerning morbidity, back-disorders result in 175 million lost workdays every year with people over 45 being the most highly affected age group.

Lumbar Anatomy

When discussing the lower back I am generally referring to the lumbar area of the spine. It contains the five lowest vertebrae and is located between the thoracic spine (middle back) and the lowest bone called the sacrum. Between each vertebra is a capsule of connective tissue (annulus fibrosus) with a soft, jellylike center (nucleus pulposus, or nucleus), called a disc. The job of the disc is to absorb shock and make the spine flexible.

The spinal cord runs through a canal (spinal canal) that is formed by the openings in each of the vertebrae. Nerves branch from the spinal cord, pass through openings (foramen) between the vertebrae, and branch to the lower body.

Traumatic Injury

Traumatic injury to the lower back comes in one of three forms: muscle strain, ligament sprain, or disc trauma. Most of us will at some point strain the muscles of our lower back by lifting improperly, having poor posture, or overworking the muscles themselves. People generally choose to self-manage a strain with over-the-counter pain relievers rather than seek professional help. Sprains are less common than strains but are often more severe.

As many as 100,000 persons are hospitalized each year due to ligament sprains of the lower back. The most serious injury to the lower back involves the disc itself. Intervertebral disc disorders result in over 400,000 hospitalizations per year.

Disc Injuries

When the disc is injured the tough fibers around it will tend to stretch and bulge. A well-known condition where a disc bulge is present is sciatica. The symptoms of sciatica include severe lower back pain with radiating pain of a burning nature from the lower back, down the outside part of the leg and ending in the big toe. This type of pain is usually debilitating. Sciatica results from a disc bulging to one side and placing pressure on a spinal nerve root. Nerve roots are attached directly to the spinal cord and are the beginning part of the nerve. The sciatic nerve begins as three separate nerve roots combine to form one long nerve that travels down the leg, branching out as it goes, and ending in the foot. When nerve roots are irritated by pressure, either from a disc bulge or from localized inflammation, they produce the symptoms of pain, numbness and/or tingling. The symptoms can be specific to a muscle in the buttock or hip, or they can traverse the length of the nerve itself.

Disc injuries can be managed quite well with non-invasive hands-on techniques like manual adjustments or vector point cranial therapy. Nutrition and at-home programs are also a significant part of recovery. Conservative care for disc injuries of the lower back, including sciatica, is used by complimentary doctors on a daily basis with excellent success. Far too often, people with disc injuries are operated on surgically. I know this is true for two reasons. 1. According to several published studies in this country and in Great Britain, conservative treatments, like the ones I use in this office, are the most effective methods of treatment for lower back pain. This means that orthopedic surgeons should be referring many of these patients to chiropractors. Instead, 2. The United States performs up to four times as many surgeries for disc problems per capita than other industrialized countries. The statistics below are for Discetomies - surgery where the disc is actually removed.

- Great Britain: 100 per 1 million persons / year
- Sweden: 200 per 1 million person / year
- Finland: 350 per 1 million persons / year
- **United States: 1,310 per 1 million persons / year**

Based on the above, it seems reasonable to ask, "If conservative care works to restore function better than other therapies including surgery, and leaves my spine intact, not removing anything from it, why would I first want to see a surgeon?"

Causes of Low Back Pain

Although it is commonly thought of as being related to an injury, there are actually over one hundred causes of lower back pain. For simplicity I have placed them into four categories:

1. *Subluxations* - Subluxation is a fancy term for the misalignment of a joint. This is what chiropractors spend most of their time correcting. When a subluxation is present there are a number of findings such as pain, swelling, redness, muscle spasm, and even neurological changes like decreased muscle strength, numbness and tingling. Subluxations can result from any type of stress: minor trauma, poor diet and emotional issues.

2. *Any Chronic Stress* – Almost any problem can be the result of any stress given enough time. That is why patients are often perplexed. They do not understand how they could suddenly have lower back pain (or any other condition) when they haven't done anything strenuous. They may not have physically over worked their back, but they have eaten a poor diet, causing toxins to build up in their tissues; they have been constipated for many years, inflaming and over working their colon; they have been taking birth control pills, severely altering normal hormonal function; they have burned the candle at both ends, not allowing their body to rest and regenerate; and so on. Chronic stress will accumulate and produce lower back pain (at the least).

3. *Severe Trauma* – This is perhaps the most easily understood cause of lower back pain. Someone bends over and picks up a fifty pound bag of fertilizer or overdoes it in the gym.

4. *Viscero-Somatic Reflexes* – This term simply means that an upset organ (viscera) produces pain of some kind in a muscle (soma) or possibly a joint. Menstrual cramps are a good example. When the ovaries and uterus are strenuously worked once a month the result is pain in the lower abdominal region. The large intestine likewise, has an intimate relationship with the lower back and therefore when irritated, will produce back pain of an achy nature. On the other hand, psycho-somatic or psycho-viscero reflexes originate within the mind from emotional stresses. They are common when people get upset or nervous and then develop symptoms in their stomach or further down the digestive tract.

Correction with Applied Kinesiology

Remember from earlier that applied kinesiology uses diagnostic muscle testing to evaluate the body's structural, chemical and emotional components. Besides the protocols I discuss in the chapter on Chronic Illness, there are a few steps specific to treating lower back pain.

1. *Test and correct the muscles of the lower back and pelvis*
2. *Realign the subluxated bones*
3. *Address nutritional / chemical stresses*
4. *Address emotional stresses*
5. *Exercises when appropriate*

The Muscles

The vertebrae of the lower back are supported by spinal ligaments and the following muscle groups:

- *Abdominal muscles support the spine from the front of the body.*
- *Iliopsoas muscles support the spine and flex the hips.*

- *Erector spinae support the back of the trunk and spine and are the major stabilizers of the spine during lifting.*

Correcting Low Back Pain

Putting bones in their proper place is just as important as balancing poor functioning muscles. There are several methods I use to help rid the body of low back pain.

1. *Pelvic blocking* – Simple triangular wedges are inserted underneath both sides of the pelvis in a therapeutic manner. This non-force procedure is extremely effective at rebalancing muscles around subluxated joints, as well as gently coaxing the misaligned bones back in place. Generally there will be a number of sore points in the muscles around a subluxated joint. After the blocks have done their work, the sore spots will be gone or greatly reduced. This process generally takes only a few minutes and is an excellent example of how a properly directed procedure can have profound effects with very little effort.

2. *De-imbrication* – An imbrication occurs when two vertebrae are jammed together. This usually only occurs on either the right or the left side of two juxtaposed vertebrae. It is commonly found when a muscle spasm is present. For instance, if a patient complains of right sided lower back muscle spasms, it is likely that these spasms have gradually forced two vertebrae together in an exaggerated manner, creating an imbrication. This problem will generally result in severe pain with difficulty standing or bending backwards. The good news is that it is easy to fix. The process of de-imbricating a patient requires a quick and properly directed traction of the leg on the side of pain. Many patients have considered this procedure a miracle cure because of the significant amount of relief obtained once performed.

3. *Vector Point Cranial Therapy* – see: SECTION I: Vector Point Cranial Therapy

4. *Manual adjustments* – see: SECTION I: Spinal Adjustments

5. *Chemical balancing* – see: SECTION I: Supplementation. There are specific chemical reactions taking place within the body whenever pain and inflammation are present. Thankfully, there are a number of herbs and supplements that can reduce these reactions, greatly aiding recovery. Likewise, if tissues such as muscles and ligaments have been strained or sprained respectively, they can benefit measurably from proper supplementation. Using applied kinesiology I test to see which nutrients will be the most beneficial for a particular patient. Proteolytic enzymes, specific B-vitamins, detoxification nutrients such as milk thistle and taurine and anti-inflammatory nutrients such as turmeric and bromelain as well as many others, can all be used therapeutically.

6. *Emotional balancing* – see: SECTION I: EMOTIONAL THERAPIES. All the parts of the body are in some way interconnected and affected by adverse stress in any of its forms. However, certain connections are stronger than others. Some emotional stresses have a greater impact on the lower back through their connections within the nervous system. For example, emotions such as vulnerability, insecurity, or feeling lost or abandoned affect the small intestine over time. The small intestine has a strong influence over the fifth lumber vertebrae – the lowest vertebrae in the back, the one most commonly involved in lower back pain. It can therefore be highly therapeutic for the patient with low back pain if emotional stresses are addressed through neuroemotional therapy.

7. *Diet* – see: SECTION II: Diet. Diet is important in the recovery of any chronic condition including lower back pain. The most important things to do are to avoid refined and processed foods such as sugar, white flour, sodas, crackers and alcohol. These foods contribute to the inflammatory state that is already present. Next, you must eat foods that are nutritious and aid in the healing process. These are organic whole foods such as fruits, vegetables, eggs, butter, meats, fish and pure water. Unless overcooked or processed, whole foods will assist in their own digestion through the nutrients and enzymes contained within them.

WEIGHT LOSS

There is an epidemic of preventable illness in our country. Currently, 64.5% of Americans are either obese or overweight (25% of Americans are obese). People are considered to be obese if they are more than 20% of their ideal weight. Ideal weight is determined with the following considerations: height, age, sex and build.

Amazingly, 6 of the top 10 causes of death are directly related to being overweight or obese. This means that almost 71% of all deaths in our country each year are related to a preventable problem. Here are some of the causes of weight gain:

- Overeating.
- Poor eating habits (high-carbohydrate, high-calorie diet).
- Lack of exercise.
- Emotional factors such as guilt, depression, and anxiety.
- Slower metabolism, which is normal with aging.
- Smoking cessation.
- Alcohol consumption.
- Primary hypothyroidism.
- Endocrine disorders including Cushing's syndrome or polycystic ovary syndrome.
- Drugs such as corticosteroids, cyproheptadine, lithium, tranquilizers, phenothiazines, and tricyclic antidepressants.

- Medications that increase fluid retention and cause edema (or the abnormal pooling of fluids in the tissues).

Americans have been deceived by food companies, advertisers, and even the government itself through the recommended food pyramid. Beyond this, urban and suburban living subject us to greater time constraints leaving less time for proper food selection and preparation; the technological age has made our tasks easier and our lives more sedentary; stresses of all kinds have increased, changing our internal chemistry and promoting fat storage rather than fat burning; and parents have passed bad habits down to their children – 1 out of 4 children are overweight or obese. You will compete against these and other obstacles as you travel on the road to health.

Having said all this, even with the cultural, social and environmental factors raised against you, you can take responsibility and act for your own good. You have a mind, an opportunity and a will. Use your mind to learn about that which is good and beneficial; use your opportunity to apply what you learn; use your will to act today and tomorrow in the wisdom that you are leading a healthy life.

I will be honest with you; it is not easy to take back control. You are, as most are, addicted to food. If you don't believe me, try avoiding sugar, bread or coffee. Food addictions can have as much power as drugs and alcohol. But the battle is not always uphill. Once you regain control, sometimes within a few weeks, you will not have the same desires you used to. If you make your entire body healthier with nutritional balancing, exercise and detoxification, you will develop a distaste for the sugar-filled foods you once enjoyed.

Healthy Weight Loss

It is important to understand that not all weight loss programs are the same. My goal is to teach you to lose weight by building a healthy body. This means overcoming three specific obstacles – what I call metabolic stumbling blocks. This can be done with the information in this book. In some cases professional help is required (see: SECTION I: Health Questionnaire).

Healthy weight loss requires a change in metabolism - the processes within the body by which energy is made available. A healthy metabolism will optimize hormonal levels like insulin and cortisol (an adrenal gland hormone), detoxify unwanted chemicals, produce abundant energy, and burn fat as its primary fuel.

3 Steps to Healthy Weight Loss

1. Remove the 3 Metabolic Stumbling Blocks
    a. Hormonal imbalances
    b. Inflammatory reactions
    c. Toxic overload

    } **H.I.T.**
2. Exercise (see: Exercise in the AT HOME section)
3. Diet (see: Diet in the AT HOME section)

Goals of Healthy Weight Loss
1. Improve overall health
    a. Maintain or increase muscle mass
    b. Develop a fat burning metabolism
    c. Reduce the risk of illness
    d. Increase energy
    e. Increase cognitive function (think better)
2. Look good

Body Mass Index
Simply reducing calories in not sufficient when H.I.T. is present and will result in unhealthy weight loss. Reducing calories may cause you to lose weight but it will overburden the body with toxins and promote muscle burning for fuel, leading to a poor Body Mass Index (BMI).

Muscle mass is perhaps the most important factor in determining how healthy we will be in our later years. You can continue to gain muscle mass well into your 60's. Healthy weight loss means burning fat without losing muscle. 20% of "thin" Americans have an unhealthy body composition. This means that even though they are thin and look fine in their clothes, they have too much fat and not enough muscle. These people are just as likely to suffer from chronic illnesses as someone who is overweight.

There are ways to measure your body mass including, bio-electric impedance testing, waist-to-hip ratio, and skin fold thickness. Your body mass index can also be calculated with the following formula:

$$\text{Weight} \div (\text{height})^2 \times 704.5$$

A BMI of 25 to 29.9 is considered overweight,
a BMI of 30 or more is considered obese.

Example: if you weighed 140lbs and were 5′2″ then your BMI is

$$(140 \div 62*62) \times 704.5 = 25.7$$

In this case, 25.7, is just within the overweight range. However, calculating BMI is not always accurate. BMI is based on human averages. Muscular people may not calculate with a good score although their ratio of muscle to fat is quite healthy. Pregnant women will also not calculate a valid score.

Example: I am 6′2″ tall and weigh 195 lbs. My BMI is

$$(195 \div 74*74) \times 704.5 = 25.1$$

This number is just inside the overweight range as well. However, I am far from overweight. In fact, most people think I am skinny. Your actual number does not matter that much, you can still use these calculations as a guide to judge improvements. If you lose fat and gain muscle your BMI will get lower. As you begin your weight loss program, use the tracking sheets in the back of this book to record your progress.

METABOLIC STUMBLING BLOCKS

Some people have a very hard time losing weight. Even if their present emotional and lifestyle factors are good the weight just does not come off. Most likely these people are storing fat because of normal metabolic process forced out of control. This can happen because someone has incurred a great deal of stress over a short period of time or more likely, a moderate degree of stress over a long period of time. Both will produce altered metabolic function and potentially lead to weight gain.

When I say stress, I mean any type of stress: structural, chemical emotional, or environmental. Any of these will produce a chemical reaction within the body that is hormonal, inflammatory or toxic. In fact, any disease you can think of has a hormonal, inflammatory or toxic component – often they have all three. That is why I place such heavy emphasis on these particular stumbling blocks. If you can control H.I.T. you will not only help reduce your weight, you will also overcome illness.

HORMONES

Hormones are a very complicated set of substances. They are directly related to every action that takes place within the body. Hormonal imbalances can produce a number of symptoms including:

- Depression / anxiety
- Water retention
- Sleeplessness
- Hot flashes
- Menstrual irregularities
- Fatigue
- Weight gain

Insulin is an important hormone. Imbalances in this hormone can be related to being overweight. Its job is to tell the cell that sugar is available for fuel in the blood stream. Under certain circumstances, this process stops working correctly resulting in a condition called Hyperinsulinemia. Hyperinsulinemia is one part of The Deadly Quartet a.k.a. *Insulin Resistance Syndrome*. The other parts are abnormal sugar (glucose) metabolism, abnormal fat (lipid) metabolism, and high blood pressure. The state of Hyperinsulinemia is directly related to the ingestion of large amounts of carbohydrates, especially the refined kind (white flour, white sugar, white rice etc.). Hyperinsulinemia (too much insulin), both in the fasting state and in response to glucose load or a meal, appears as one of the first major abnormalities of obesity.

Most obese people eat the same number of calories at meal times as non-obese people. However, obese people tend to snack on carbohydrate foods in the evening, adding an additional 800 calories to their otherwise normal diet. Since it takes approximately 3500 calories to make one pound of fat, eating an additional 800 calories at night could mean gaining 1 pound of body fat every 4 to 5 days, or as much as 90 pounds each year.

When insulin resistance exists, the body attempts to correct itself by secreting more insulin from the pancreas. Eventually, this compensatory action cannot continue and results in the development of Type II, or non-insulin dependent diabetes. It is not clear how insulin resistance contributes to the presence of high blood pressure, but it is clear that the high insulin levels resulting from insulin resistance contribute to abnormalities in blood lipids such as cholesterol and triglycerides.

High insulin levels from refined food intake are also related to depression, though the mechanisms are not fully understood. A 2002 University of Texas Southwestern Medical Center survey of six countries found that those populations with higher per capita refined sugar consumption corresponded with higher rates of depression.

The presence of any of the four factors of Insulin Resistance Syndrome creates a significant risk for chronic illness. In combination or with other risk factors such as a sedentary lifestyle, high stress, smoking, and genetic predisposition, the risk becomes exponential. For instance, the risk for heart attack is increased 2.5 times when diabetes or high blood pressure is present. When both diabetes and high blood pressure are present, the risk is increased 8 times. An abnormal lipid profile increases the risk 16 times; and when abnormal lipid levels were present with high blood pressure and/or diabetes, the risk for a heart attack increases 20 times.

INFLAMMATION

Inflammation is a bodily response to an injury or health condition that is characterized by pain, swelling, and a loss of mobility. The inflammatory process is quite complex and is characterized by (1) vasodilatation (enlargement) of the local blood vessels causing an increase in blood flow, (2) increased permeability of the small blood vessels (capillaries) resulting in large quantities of fluid leaky into the spaces between the tissues and cells, (3) clotting of the fluid in the inflamed area due to the presence of a substance called fibrinogen, (4) migration of large numbers of monocytes and granulocytes (white blood cells that help eliminate the damaged tissue), and (5) swelling of the injured tissue cells. These reactions are the result of chemical substances such as histamine, bradykinin, serotonin, and prostaglandins (see: COMMON CHRONIC CONDITIONS: Pain).

Inflammatory processes can be part of a number of conditions including:

- Joint pain (arthritis)
- Muscle pain (myositis)
- Headaches
- Swelling (edema)
- Digestive irregularities (colitis, gastritis)
- Auto-immune diseases (Rheumatoid arthritis)
- Weight loss or gain

When inflammation is present in a tissue for a long period of time another significant reaction can take place on a cellular level called the alarm state. The alarm state alters the normal function within every cell causing *fat storage* and the breakdown of protein for fuel (catabolism). Unless the alarm state is reversed, losing weight is nearly impossible. I discuss some natural anti-inflammatory substances in SECTION III: Health Cabinet.

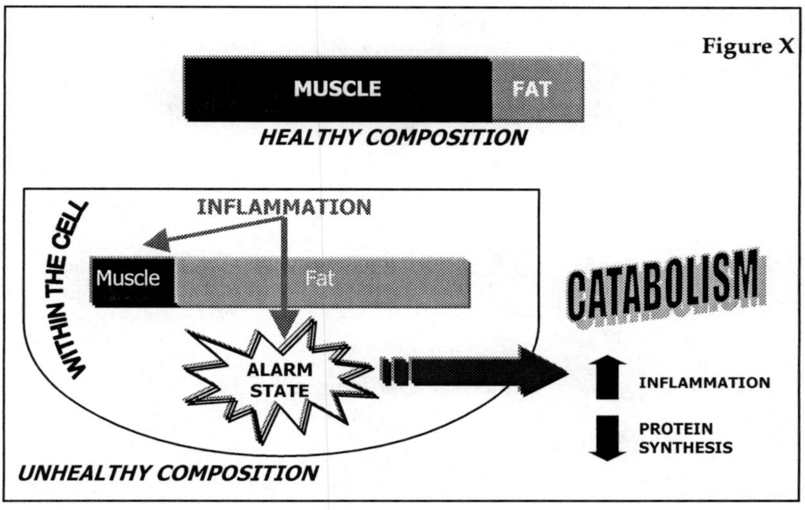

TOXICITY

Toxicity is the "T" in H.I.T. and is the most prevalent of the metabolic stumbling blocks. Toxicity is an unhealthy state of toxic buildup. Toxins are found everywhere and can be almost anything. There is little chance of escape. Look at these statistics in the United States for example.

- There are currently 400 different pesticides types available for use.
- 2.5 billion pounds of pesticides are used on croplands, forests, lawns, & fields.
- 24.6 million tons of antibiotics are fed to livestock.
- 750,000 dairy cows are injected with growth hormone.
- Over 80 million acres of genetically engineered crops are presently under cultivation. The long-term effects of these foods are as yet undetermined.

Toxic Food

These statistics have to do with what happens to food before it is prepared to eat. Food preparation - how it is cooked or processed – may produce toxins. Also, food additives such as monosodium glutamate (msg) may be toxic as well. The average American eats about 125 pounds of additives and 175 pounds of sugar per year.

Foods most contaminated with pesticides:

▪ Apples	▪ Apricots
▪ Bell peppers	▪ Celery
▪ Chilean grapes	▪ Cucumbers
▪ Green beans	▪ Mexican cantaloupe
▪ Peaches	▪ Spinach
▪ Strawberries	▪ U.S. Cherries

Figure XI

Toxic Water

The Environmental Protection Agency monitors our drinking water for safe levels of microorganisms, disinfectants, disinfectant by-products, inorganic chemicals, organic chemicals, and radionuclides. In 2002, approximately 260 millions pounds of chemicals were released into surface waters. Since the EPA measures for safe levels and not merely for the presence of toxic substances, you know that the water you consume is already contaminated to some extent. Any water filter is a good idea.

Toxic Air

Air quality has been improving in this country. Despite this positive trend, 170 million tons of air emissions are released into the atmosphere annually. These released agents are more potential toxins that must be processed by the body.

You may have heard the name, "free radicals." These are chemicals produced under normal circumstances inside a cell every time oxygen is used for energy. The problem is not that they exist, rather that the neutralizing agents, called anti-oxidants, are no longer plentiful. Anti-oxidants can be any of a number of compounds including vitamins and minerals. When the body's nutritional reserves cannot keep up with demand then damage from free radicals occurs - making even the air you breathe dangerous to your health. The average person breathes 3,400 gallons of air each day. Depending upon your current state of health, even clean air may be a source of harm.

Other Sources

I have already mentioned the toxic sources from what we eat, drink and breathe. There are also other toxins that we voluntarily ingest such as medications, low quality supplements, birth control pills, recreational and illegal drugs.

Symptoms of Toxicity

Toxins accumulate in the body either because of too much exposure, or because the body is not adequately processing and eliminating them. Here are only a few of the symptoms of toxicity:

- Fatigue
- Fibromyalgia
- Sleep disturbance
- GI distress
- Headaches
- Allergy symptoms
- Confusion
- Hormonal imbalances

Toxic Effects

Toxins within the body create havoc in a number of ways. Many of the pesticides that are eventually dumped into our rivers have estrogenic effects. This means that they act like estrogen hormones in your body, preventing proper hormonal function and production. They also affect the receptor sites where hormones bind, further altering function. It is believed that these estrogenic compounds are responsible in part for the current explosion in hormone cancers, increased hypothyroidism, early female puberty; low sperm counts in males and the loss of libido of both sexes.

These estrogenic effects take their toll on animals as well. Lake Apopka in Florida, an intensely toxic lake full of pesticides, produced hermaphroditic fish and markedly de-masculinized male alligators. The next generation of alligators born at the lake was 100% female.

Besides affecting hormones, toxins also create inflammation and tissue fatigue. So we see that the metabolic stumbling blocks feed off of one another in a vicious cycle of regressive health.

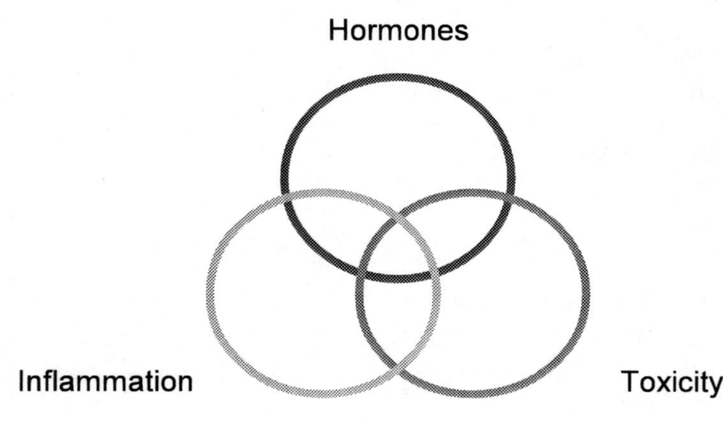

Figure XI

To get an idea of your current level of toxicity please take the toxicity self test in the back of the book or visit my website www.choosehealth.net and click on Toxicity Self Test.

Complicating Factors to Weight Loss

As if the metabolic stumbling blocks were not enough, there are other immune system burdens that make weight loss difficult. I always check patients for food allergies. When present, food allergies can lead to a number of digestive difficulties including leaky gut syndrome – an inflammatory condition of the gut where food and nutrients are not properly absorbed.

Food allergies can be either genetic or acquired. Most likely they are acquired; the result of a long-term bad diet and poor lifestyle factors. There is a direct relationship between the health of the digestive system and the prevalence of food allergies. There is also a direct relationship between the health of the digestive system and the health of the body. Food is the primary agent for microorganisms and poisons that could potentially harm the body. It is therefore not surprising to discover that up to 70% of the immune system is located in the linings of the intestines.

Correcting H.I.T.

There are three steps to losing weight: control H.I.T., eat a proper diet, and exercise. Proper diet and exercise will themselves help correct H.I.T. and are discussed in their own respective sections. Beyond that I use my chronic illness protocol (see: Section I, Chronic Illness). This mean that I desensitize discovered food allergens, aggressively prescribe healing nutrients, rebalance the body's structure with hands-on therapies, remove or reduce neuroemotional complexes, and generally support the patient through this important transformation. In other words, I use a whole person approach.

Therapeutic Supplementation

I use a number of different nutritional supplements depending upon the patient's individual needs. If applicable however, I like to use a product called MediClear® from Thorne Research. It is a rice-based protein powder that contains many agents in highly absorbable forms. On the label it says that it is designed to "reduce inflammation, aid in detoxification, and reduce the effects of allergies". You can see why I like it. Generally I have the patient start slow (1/2 – 1 scoop at meal time) and increase it from there. I want to limit the adverse effects of aggressive detoxification (see: SECTION III, Detoxification). This will help with compliance and long-term success.

AT HOME

SECTION III

DIET & FOODS

The human body is made up of countless numbers of chemicals, each designed to carry out a specific function for the benefit of the body as a whole. The presence of essential chemicals means a better chance for vibrant health, while the absence of essential chemicals means a better chance for disease. This is important for our discussion on diet because the required chemicals (nutrients) we need for health can only come from what we eat.

From a scientific viewpoint we have learned that when the cells of our body die and new cells are formed, the materials needed to make those tissues come from the macro and micronutrients in our diet. Macronutrients include three main building blocks: carbohydrates, proteins and fats. The micronutrients include: minerals, vitamins, enzymes and thousands of other co-factors whose job is to regulate the activity of the macronutrients. It is essential that these nutrients be of high quality. If you are not careful about the type and quality of food you eat, your poor diet will result in poor or absent nutrients and a greater potential for disease.

It has taken a long time, but the erroneous idea that diet has little to do with the prevention or elimination of disease, is now beginning to slowly fade. Science repeatedly confirms what those with some common sense have known all along: good diets make you healthy, while bad diets eventually cause illness.

In my own practice, I have regularly used diet modification and nutritional measures to greatly relieve or eliminate many chronic ailments. I use very simple and easy to follow guidelines discussed at the end of this chapter. These guidelines plus an understanding of the basics of the macronutrients will equip you to make healthier food choices.

CARBOHYDRATES

Carbohydrates come mostly from plant sources. When broken down into their most basic parts (sugars) they become an important fuel for many tissues within the body. This means that they are an essential part of a healthy diet.

Carbohydrates are classified according to their molecular structure. There are three types: simple carbohydrates (sugars), complex carbohydrates (starches) and plant fibers (cellulose, hemicellulose and pectin). Simple carbohydrates are the ones that do the most harm. In the chapter on Weight Loss, I discuss how eating too many simple carbohydrates places a heavy burden on the hormonal tissues responsible for regulating blood sugar levels and will eventually lead to carbohydrate intolerance (insulin resistance).

Simple carbohydrates include: monosaccharides, which contain only a single sugar and oligosaccharides, which are a combination of two or more monosaccharides. The complex carbohydrates are called polysaccharides because they are made up of many simple sugars.

Simple Carbohydrates (Monosaccharides)	
Glucose (a.k.a. Dextrose, corn sugar, grape sugar) **Fructose**	Glucose is the form of carbohydrate found circulating in the blood. Because glucose is absorbed directly into the blood stream when ingested creating a dramatic insulin response, it should be limited in the diet. Fructose is a monosaccharide that is absorbed at half the rate of glucose. It is found in honey, ripe fruit and some vegetables (corn).
Simple Carbohydrates (Oligosaccharides)	
Sucrose, Sugar cane, Sugar beets, Molasses,	Sucrose is common table sugar. Although it is a simple carbohydrate just like the others listed, it is far less healthy. The others are "complete", that is, they are combined with vitamins,

Maple sugar, Sorghum	minerals, enzymes and fibers. The effect is better absorption and regulation within the body. Sucrose has none of these nutrients.
Simple Carbohydrates (Others)	
Lactose	Lactose from milk is a disaccharide, containing one molecule of glucose and one molecule of galactose. Lactose is a good food source if the dairy has been properly prepared (see: Preparing Foods) and if you have the enzyme lactase, needed to break down lactose. 20% of White and 80% of Black children do not have this important enzyme.
Complex Carbohydrates (digestible)	
Starch, Dextrin, Glycogen	Although composed of sugar, these are usually not sweet tasting. Glycogen is synthesized in the liver and is the stored fuel used for immediate energy. Glycogen is rapidly used up under extreme activities like sprinting or heavy weight lifting.
Complex Carbohydrates (indigestible) - Fiber	
<u>Soluble:</u> pectins, gums & mucilages **<u>Insoluble:</u> cellulose and hemicellulose.**	Plants contain mixtures of fibers; some that dissolve in water (soluble) and some that don't (insoluble). Cellulose, an indigestible fiber, represents more than 1/3 of the total organic material produced by plants. Soluble fiber can help lower cholesterol, while the non-soluble fiber is good for adding bulk to the intestinal contents, which aids in elimination.

Figure XII

FATS

When discussing the topic of fats, I am really talking about a class of compounds called lipids. These include triglycerides, phospholipids, cholesterol, prostaglandins and fatty acids. Lipids play many important roles in the body. They are part of the membrane structure of all cells and can be metabolized for an energy source or stored as fat. However, most of the time they are converted into substances called prostaglandins.

PROSTAGLANDINS

Prostaglandins (PG) are hormone-like substances. There are 3 main groups (PG1, PG2, and PG3), each converted from three different categories or "families" of fats. In figure XIV you see that PG2 has inflammatory qualities, whereas PG1 and PG3 have anti-inflammatory qualities. That PG2 is inflammatory does not necessarily mean that it is bad. In fact, when it is present in proportion to the other prostaglandins, it is highly beneficial. However, under certain conditions such as vitamin deficiencies, eating too many fats from the PG2 family and regular ingestion of hydrogenated fats, the body by default produces more PG2 than PG1 or PG3. The net effect is an imbalance in the levels of prostaglandins and a systemic inflammatory process.

SATURATD FATS

As I discuss in the chapter, Cholesterol, some cultures around the world have diets historically high in saturated fat but DO NOT have heart disease like we do in America. In some cases, like the Eskimos of North America or the Masai tribes of Africa, despite extremely high dietary levels of meat and saturated fat, heart disease is non-existent. This reality runs countercurrent to what we are told regularly by most doctors who say that saturated fat is the primary reason for heart disease and clogged arteries. When they say saturated fat, they generally mean animal fat. However, saturated fat is found in many sources including: coconut oil, palm oil, cottonseed oil and a variety of nuts. Confusing the issue further is the fact that most of the fat found in clogged arteries is poly<u>unsaturated</u>. This means it did not come from the saturated fats found in animal or vegetable products. Polyunsaturated fats tend to become oxidized or rancid when exposed to heat through cooking. Excess polyunsaturated oils like corn, soy, safflower and canola oils, have been shown to cause several diseases including:

heart disease, immune system dysfunction, organ damage, digestive disorders, depressed learning ability, impaired growth, and weight gain.

Saturated fats do have some know detrimental effects such as blocking delta-6-desaturase, an enzyme that helps convert non-animal fats into PG1 and PG3 (the anti-inflammatory prostaglandins). They can also raise cholesterol, produce autoimmune diseases, and lead to heart attack and stroke; but only when the ratio of saturated fat to unsaturated fat is too high. When the ratio is balanced the detrimental effects are greatly minimized. So what is the proper ratio? There is no hard and fast rule because genetics seem to have a strong influence. Some people can eat a great deal of saturated fat without endangering their health. However, there is one type of fat responsible for lipid-related diseases that should be avoided by everyone.

HYDROGENATED FATS

Hydrogenated oils, partially hydrogenated oils, or trans-fats, are all processed fats. This means that they have been altered from their original form by injection with hydrogen, in order to increase "freshness" and shelf life. Most of the foods you see in the middle isles of the grocery store, the ones that come in boxes or bags and can sit in the shelf for months at a time, contain high amounts of hydrogenated oils. These include cereals, crackers, cookies, baked foods, prebaked foods, chips, snack bars, breakfast bars, frozen foods and more.

Hydrogenated oils cause a host of problems:

- Interfere with the normal conversion of fats to PG1 and PG3.
- Cause an increase in the production of PG2.
- Block the normal conversion of cholesterol in the liver leading to elevated cholesterol levels.
- They become part of the building blocks of our cells, displacing desired materials and disrupting cellular function.

EATING FATS

As a general rule, to get the right ratio of fats from your diet, you should eat foods high in omega 3 fats such as fish and flax seed, eat moderate amounts of animal fats, reduce or eliminate heated polyunsaturated fats, and eliminate hydrogenated oils.

PROSTA-GLANDIN	PG1 (anti-inflammatory)	PG2 (inflammatory)	PG3 (anti-inflammatory)
	Omega-6 Fats	**Animal Fats (saturated)**	**Omega-3 Fats**
Created From	Safflower, corn, peanut, almond, canola, soy, cottonseed, black currant seed oil, primrose oil, borage oil, wheat germ oil	Butter, cream, milk, cheese, meat, egg yolks, shellfish.	Fish oil, EPA, flaxseed oil, linseed oil, walnut oil, sesame seed oil, leafy greens, beans.
Increased With	Delta-6-desaturase, moderate alcohol, niacin, B6, zinc, magnesium, low dose vitamin E (<400iu), aerobic exercise.	Insulin and aging, strenuous activity, low protein and possibly fiber.	Delta-6-desaturase, vitamin C, low dose vitamin E (<400iu), EPA, B6, zinc, magnesium.
Inhibited By	Hydrogenated fats, saturated fats, aspirin (NSAIDS), aspartame, steroids, high dose ethyl alcohol, food additives, high dose vitamin E (>400iu).	Delta-6-desaturase (D-6-D) Decreased by: EPA, raw sesame oil, aspirin (NSAIDS), high dose vitamin E (>400iu).	Hydrogenated fats, saturated fats, aspirin (NSAIDS), aspartame, steroids, ethyl alcohol, food additives, high dose vitamin E (>400iu).

Figure XIII

PROTEINS

Proteins make up a large portion of our bones, muscles, organs, teeth, skin, nails and hair. They are necessary for the repair and rebuilding of all body tissues. Proteins are made up of amino acids. Scientists are currently aware of twenty two different types of amino acids, eight of which are essential. This means that they must be supplied by the diet. The non-essential amino acids can be manufactured by the body. The body does have a reserve capacity for the essential amino acids and other nutrients so that when the diet is incomplete, the body can draw from its reserves.

Protein comes from a variety of sources. Meats, fish, eggs, and chicken are the most common examples. However, seeds, nuts, legumes and beans also contain concentrated amounts. It is my opinion that protein should be consumed in all of its forms. However, because of the protein available in non-animal products, for health reasons and reasons of conscience many have decided to turn to vegetarianism.

Proponents of vegetarianism are quick to tout the health benefits from eating a non-meat die such as a reduced incidence of heart disease, breast and prostate cancers. However, each of these outcomes can also be achieved even when meat is eaten. In general, I do not advocate strict vegetarianism. For some it may be acceptable, but I have often seen vegetarian patients who were slow to recover from their aliments because of low amounts of dense animal proteins. On my insistence, they reluctantly agreed to include more of these proteins in their diet and not surprisingly, their health improves.

I believe that metabolic individuality (genetics) is perhaps the greatest consideration when attempting to determine if meat sources of protein are satisfactory. In my own case, while in chiropractic college, I began a popular diet that promoted high raw fruit and vegetable consumption with very little meat consumption. It almost killed me. I have never been that sick or frail in my life. It is true that there were other stressful factors that contributed to my near demise such as completing my training, deciding where to practice, opening an office and so on. Yet, presently my stress is at times no less; but having learned that my body requires considerable amounts of dense protein, I function at a much higher level without succumbing to sickness. I have seen similar changes with numerous patients when a personalized diet was introduced. It has become my goal with any treatment program to find those key elements that relate specifically to each patient.

PROPER PROTEIN DIGESTION

Proteins begin digestion in the acid environment of the stomach. Then in the small intestine, enzymes from the pancreas complete the process. Although proteins are digested differently than fats and carbohydrates, inadequate digestion of all three macronutrients occurs if:

- There is not enough hydrochloric acid in the stomach.
- There are inadequate enzymes from the pancreas.
- The small intestine is irritated and inflamed (leaky gut).
- Complimentary nutrients are not available for complete processing.
- Any combination of the above.

LISTENING TO YOUR BODY

With the basics of macronutrients covered, here now are some practical steps to eating healthy. As you begin adding these principles of eating into your life, you must pay attention to one very important component: listening to your body. In the Philosophy chapter, I discussed how the body is always adapting to and resisting stress. Food is often a stress. That is because people's food choices are not always the best. Listening to your body simply means becoming aware of any changes that occur while under stress, or after eating food. These signals indicate that something is wrong.

Food has several purposes. One of these is to reinvigorate us. In other words, we should notice a surge of energy immediately after eating healthy food. If this is not so, it may be a clue. Keep in mind no single food is perfect for everyone. It is not uncommon for foods, even "healthy" foods, to cause problems in different people. It is important therefore, to discern between those foods that react well with your body and those that do not.

The technique is simple. Think about how your body feels before you eat. Are you currently experiencing any of the problems in the list below? If the answer is yes, put that information in your memory bank, then go ahead and eat.

- Bloating
- Burping (the food you taste is probably the provocative one)
- Dizziness
- Fatigue / sleepiness
- Gas
- Headache
- Increased heart rate
- Intestinal gurgling
- Lightheadedness
- Mucous in the throat
- Stiff muscles
- Stuffiness in the head or sinuses
- Tight joints
- Weakness

After you have eaten and within the next hour or so, analyze yourself again. Do you now experience any of the above symptoms? Did the ones you had before get any worse? If so, you can be sure that your body has a problem with one or more of the foods you just ate.

This technique will get easier the longer you eat healthfully. Practice is also important. The more you practice this technique, the easier it is to "hear" the right information. Unfortunately, most people have ignored their body's responses for so long that they have lost the ability to recognize the warning signals. For instance, if you just finished eating a double fudge brownie and a scoop of vanilla ice cream with caramel sauce and feel just fine, chances are you've lost some ability to hear. With time, you will get the hang of it. Due to the low nutrient and high chemical content of most store bought and restaurant foods, you might be surprised at just how many foods your body finds offensive.

Below are the two lists I give to patients with regards to eating. They are principles, not a strict diet plan, though that may be required in certain instances.

BUILDING YOUR IMMUNE SYSTEM

1. Do not over eat! This is perhaps the most important guideline. As I observe those who live long and healthy lives, no matter how they eat they usually have one thing in common: they do not over eat. Consequently, these folks are often thin. They eat desserts and other less than optimal foods but only in small amounts.

2. Eat a wide variety. Of the 4,000 or so edible plants that have fed people for thousands of years, only 150 are widely cultivated today and just three of them provide 60% of the world's food. Allergies often result from eating too much of the same food – even a healthy food. I have had to take patients off of good foods because over time, they were creating problems. I had a patient who ate basically the same thing everyday. She was complaining of a skin lesion on her leg that would not go away despite considerable attention. I questioned her about her diet and was not surprised to discover that she daily ate the same handful of things. I had her bring in some samples of those foods. Applied kinesiology testing clearly showed that she was reactive to Brazil nuts and a freshly made "healthy" juice, both of which she had eaten everyday for the last 7 years.

3. Eat whole, natural foods. Whole foods are simply foods that are naturally complete. They can be picked from a tree, pulled out of the ground, or cultivated from animals. Whole foods contain chemicals within themselves that aid in their own digestion. They also contain a great number of nutrients. Fruits, vegetables, eggs, butter, some cheese, and organic meats are all examples.

4. Eat foods that will spoil (but eat them before they do). Most of the foods in the center isles of the grocery store can stay on the shelf for months at a time and still taste fresh. This is because of the many food preservatives and hydrogenated oils. On average, people in America eat 124 pounds of preservatives per year.

5. Eat naturally raised meats. The hormones and antibiotics used in making animals big and fat are beginning to take their toll. In 2002, 750,000 cows were injected with bovine

growth hormone. Hormones in beef and other meats are causing unwanted changes in people including very early menarche in girls.

6. Eat whole, naturally produced milk products (not milk by itself, unless raw) from pasture-fed cows, preferably raw and/or fermented. Milk is also full of hormones and antibiotics. It is also a highly processed food. Instead of milk eat whole yogurt, cultured butter, whole cheeses and fresh and sour cream. See SECTION IV: Resources.

7. Use traditional fats and oils. These include butter and other animal fats, extra virgin olive oil, expeller expressed sesame and flax oil and the tropical oils—coconut and palm.

8. Eat fresh fruits and vegetables, preferably organic, in salads and soups. Raw or lightly steamed is ideal.

9. Use whole grains and nuts. Prepare them by soaking, sprouting or sour leavening to neutralize harmful and hard-to-digest agents.

10. Prepare homemade meat stocks. Use the bones of chicken, beef, lamb or fish and use the stock liberally in soups and sauces.

11. Use filtered water for cooking and drinking. Our water is heavily contaminated with chemicals. This is good for killing microorganisms but bad for our bodies.

12. Use unrefined Celtic sea salt. Believe it or not, I have had several patients who needed to have salt added to their diet. The sodium found in natural salt greatly assists the adrenal glands when they are overworked.

13. Make your own condiments. Salad dressing can be made using raw vinegar, extra virgin olive oil and expeller expressed flax oil. Condiments are a high source of artificial colorings and preservatives.

14. Use natural sweeteners in moderation. These include raw honey, maple syrup, dehydrated cane sugar juice and stevia powder. Stevia now comes in convenient packs that

can be added to an herbal tea or mixed up in a healthy shake.

15. Cook only in stainless steel, cast iron, glass or good quality enamel. Aluminum cookware is easily compromised when heated leading to the release of aluminum and other metals into the food. The same is true for copper.

BREAKING YOUR IMMUNE SYSTEM

1. Avoid highly refined foods like white flour, white flour products and white rice. This also includes sweeteners such as sugar, dextrose, glucose and high fructose corn syrup. Americans eat approximately 170 pounds of sugar per year. These are not just empty calorie foods, they are negative calorie foods. This means that they require nutrients and additional energy from your body in order to be digested properly. This type of eating will take its toll quickly.
2. Avoid pasteurized milk. Milk is difficult to digest and one of the most common foods I have to remove from patient's diets. See SECTION IV: Preparing Foods.
3. Avoid all hydrogenated or partially hydrogenated fats and oils. See SECTION III: Common Chronic Conditions: Cholesterol
4. Avoid all vegetable oils made from soy, corn, safflower, canola or cottonseed. These all contain high amounts of omega 6 fats. In our society there is a great imbalance of essential fatty acids. We need more omega 3 fats that come from fish or flax seeds.
5. Limit soy products. Soybeans are high in substances called phytates, which block the absorption of essential minerals like iron. They are also enzyme inhibitors unless properly prepared by soaking in water. This means that certain proteins will not be digested properly - another cause of allergic reactions. Soybeans are best used fermented in products like *miso, natto,* and *tempeh.* Tofu is high in phytates. It should be eaten in small amounts and not as a substitute for meat. The same goes for soymilk, which consumed regularly, may lead to mineral deficiencies. The most alarming thing concerning soy and soy products are the high levels of phytoestrogens (see: Common Chronic Conditions: Women Health). These substances mimic human hormones. This can often lead to disrupted endocrine gland function. For this reason, I often counsel mothers to reduce or eliminate the amount of soy given to their pre-pubescent children.

6. Avoid artificial food additives, especially MSG, hydrolyzed vegetable protein and aspartame, which are neurotoxins. Most soups, sauces and broth mixes and commercial condiments contain MSG, even if not so labeled.
7. Avoid caffeine-containing beverages such as coffee, tea and soft drinks. Caffeine causes many problems including: addiction, over-working the adrenal glands and reducing calcium in the bones.
8. Avoid canned, sprayed, waxed, bioengineered or irradiated fruits and vegetables. These processes are designed to preserve the shelf life or speed the ripening of the food.
9. Avoid highly processed luncheon meats and sausage containing nitrites and other additives.
10. Avoid rancid and improperly prepared seeds, nuts and grains found in granolas, quick-rise breads and extruded breakfast cereals, as they block mineral absorption and cause intestinal distress.
11. Avoid synthetic vitamins and foods containing them. I am no longer amazed at the success of advertisers. For years they have been deceiving the public. Cereals promoted to children are perhaps one of the worst foods available. However, it never fails, at some point during the commercial you will be told how this product is fortified with vitamins and mineral; it contains natural fruit juices; is that a part of a healthy breakfast etc. What they don't tell you is the vitamins they use are synthetic and highly processed and therefore of little or no value to the body. They also don't tell you that their cereal is loaded with hydrogenated fats and oils; that it could sit on the shelf for four months and that as a whole it has next to no health value at all.
12. Do not eat commercially processed foods such as cookies, cakes, crackers, TV dinners, soft drinks, packaged sauce mixes, etc.
13. Do not use polyunsaturated oils for cooking, sautéing or baking. This means avoid fried foods. The high heat causes the fats to turn rancid, removing potential health benefits.

DETOXIFICATION

Detoxification is simply a term that means to get rid of toxins. It is perhaps the most essential practice of any health care regime. Detoxification is such an important process that most of our tissues participate in it, and all of our tissues are dependent upon it.

Contraindications:
In this chapter I provide some of my recommendations for detoxification. Although everyone needs to detoxify, some people need special consideration. If you are or have any of the following, consult a doctor knowledgeable in nutrition and detoxification protocols before starting:

- Cancer
- Diabetes
- Hypoglycemia
- Insulin insensitivity
- Intestinal yeast
- Obese
- All forms of Irritable bowel disease
- Women who are pregnant
- Nursing moms

HOW DO I BECOME TOXIC?

Today we are exposed to more chemicals and pollutants than in any previous generation. According to the book, *An Alternative Medicine Definitive Guide to Cancer*, "70 million Americans live in areas that exceed smog standards; most municipal drinking water contains over 700 chemicals, including excessive levels of lead. Some 3,000 chemicals are added to the food supply and as many as 10,000 chemicals, in the form of solvents, emulsifiers, and preservatives, are used in food processing and storage, which can remain in the body for years."

The reason toxins are stored in the body is a matter of efficiency. The resources allocated for detoxification are numerous and redundant, but they are still finite. If more toxins come in to the body than can be processed at any given moment, then the body must store them. Storing toxins is much less harmful than allowing them to float freely in our blood. Fat and muscle are typically the storage tissues of choice. Eventually however, if this toxin accumulation continues, the immune system suffers and the body will manifest the symptoms of toxicity. Any of the following are possible with toxicity:

- Broad mood swings
- Kidney dysfunction
- Multiple chemical sensitivities
- Abnormal pregnancy
- Contact dermatitis
- Headaches
- Cancer
- Memory loss
- Chronic fatigue syndrome
- Recurrent yeast infections
- Muscle weakness
- Unusual response to medications or supplements
- Fatigue
- Fertility problems
- Fibromyalgia
- Immune system depression
- Learning disorders
- Mineral imbalances
- Panic attacks
- Parkinson's disease
- Tinnitus
- Increasing sensitivity to strong smells
- Worsening of symptoms after anesthesia or pregnancy

WHAT SHOULD I EXPECT?

Detoxification is not fun and often, it is not easy. When done incorrectly, it can be downright awful. If the detoxification tissues are not ready to process and eliminate, you may feel badly or even get sick. Headaches, nausea, dizziness, colds, and other less than desirable symptoms are all possible during detoxification. You may ask, "If detoxification is so bad, why do it?" We have to remember something very important: Toxins are poisons. The body did the right thing by storing them but it makes no sense to keep them around any longer. The prudent thing to do is to get rid of them in a comfortable and effective way.

GETTING STARTED

Detoxification programs are numerous. This is a positive sign; it means that people recognize the benefit of cleansing toxic tissues. Unfortunately, these programs are becoming burdensome, expensive and time consuming. I have tried to simplify the process by providing both general and specific guidelines. Be diligent; remember that many of you are sick because you are toxic!

Just like controlling stress, detoxification is improved in one of two ways: reduce the number of toxins coming in, and/or increase your body's ability to remove toxins by improving the function of the detoxification tissues. Here is a list of the tools you may use to help do both.

REMOVE TOXINS:	INCREASE FUNCTION:
Diet	Exercise/ Massage
Stress Reduction	Colon Cleanse
Supplementation	Liver Cleanse
Water Purification	Kidney Cleanse
Air Purification	Skin Brushing
	Fasting

The best detoxification program would incorporate as many of the above as possible. Some should be done daily for a short time period, while others should be done forever. For most people, detoxification should be an annual or semi-annual routine.

The time spent detoxifying is related to the degree of toxicity. The more toxic, the more time needed to detoxify. If you are just getting started and are not chronically ill, try these procedures for three days. If you are chronically ill, you need to detoxify for many days, ten at least, before stopping. Be cautious. The more sick you are before starting a detoxification program, the more likely you are to experience moderate to severe side effects.

SUPPLEMENTS

If you are a beginner with detoxification you must also take some supportive supplements. This is very important. When you begin to detoxify, your body will release toxins that have been stored in your tissues for who knows how long. This is not always a pleasant experience. The right supplements will help significantly. Here is a list of supplements that assist in detoxification and many other helpful processes.

- Enzymes - Digestive distress is perhaps the most common secondary complaint among my patients. Enzymes are essential in aiding the digestive process. They also take part in *every* process in the body. All patients benefit from enzymes. I often use plant enzymes because they act in a wider pH range, making them effective throughout the entire digestive tract.
- Probiotics (bacteria) - Your body is home to over 400 types of bacteria, most of which are essential to health. Products like acidophillus, bifidobacillus, and lactobacillus are used to replenish lost bacteria in the gut. For those with Candida or Irritable Bowel Syndrome, probiotics are a must.
- Essential fatty acids (EFA's) - Fats are one of the most misunderstood macronutrients of our day, yet without them we would perish. Trans-fats like shortening and margarine are responsible for the ever-increasing rates of heart disease and high cholesterol. Eating good quality fats is a must.
- Anti-oxidants - (vitamins A, C, E, selenium, SOD, phytochemicals etc.). Doctors are learning more about antioxidants and their free radical stopping power. Free radicals are involved in every known degenerative and disease process. They cause damage through a process called oxidation (rusted metal is oxidized metal). Many toxic chemicals will be released during the detoxification process and the likelihood of oxidation is very high. Anti-oxidants are used to stop them.

- L-Glutamine powder – This is an amino acid, one of the builders of protein, and is used as a primary fuel source for the cells of the small intestine. Healing an irritated gut lining is foundational to overall health.
- Cayenne Pepper – This 'miracle' herb is good for all sorts of aliments especially digestive and circulatory complaints. The fresher and hotter, the better.
- Psyllium husk – A good bulking agent for assisting in colon cleansing.
- MediClear™ - This is a rice protein based meal-replacement powder. It is full of all sorts of ingredients to help detoxify tissues, reduce inflammation and reduce allergic reactions. I often use it as part of a weight loss program with good success.

EXERCISE

See: SECTION III: Exercise

Because of its importance not only in detoxification, but also in every process that occurs in our cells, exercise has been given its own chapter. It should not merely be part of a detoxification program, but a part of everyday life.

COLON CLEANSING

60-70% of our body's immune system is located within the linings of the intestines. This means that when the colon is inflamed, clogged or otherwise not functioning properly, neither is the immune system. If the colon is kept healthy, sickness is rarely an issue. Conversely, when we are sick, cleaning the colon will make us healthier. Since the colon is responsible for digesting and eliminating foods, the first step in colon cleansing is a clean diet.

Everyone should be sure that their colon is free from impaction and unwanted waste products. Below are the basic steps I recommend for colon health and repair. Generally speaking, if you are having less than 1 bowel movement per day, you are constipated. Steps 1 and 2 will help. If you are having less than 1 bowel movement every few days, then enemas and colonics are a must. These steps are progressive. Do not plan on doing steps 3 and 4 while skipping steps 1 and 2. None of the aids in colon cleansing will be of much long-term benefit if the diet is poor.

While cleansing your colon, if you notice that you are experiencing an uncomfortable amount of bloating or gas, eat some fresh peppermint (1 ounce with meals). Also, be sure to drink 48-64 ounces of filtered water each day.

1. My recommended diet (see: SECTION IV: Diet)

2. Supplements:

- Probiotics – Friendly bacteria, 3-6 capsules per day.
- L-Glutamine powder – 1 tablespoon 3X per day.
- Cayenne Pepper – 1 rounded teaspoon in juice or water, 3X per day.
- Psyllium husk – Begin with 1 teaspoon in water per day. Gradually increase to 3 teaspoons per day. Do not take psyllium husk with your supplements, as the fiber will reduce effectiveness.

3. Enemas:

Using liquid to loosen and assist in waste removal within the colon has proven beneficial for hundreds of years. An enema bag may be purchased at any drug store. Be careful not to allow the liquid to enter the colon too rapidly, or cramping and discomfort may result. Lie on your left side as the fluid is being dispensed. Hold the fluids for fifteen minutes and then release them while seated on the toilet. Wait a few minutes to make sure that all waste material is evacuated.

- Coffee – Brew organic caffeinated coffee, and then let it cool to body temperature before delivery via an enema bag. Coffee contains choleretics, which increase the excretion of bile from the gall bladder. This enema also aids in the second phase of liver detoxification. Coffee enemas are recognized in the medical literature and may be safely used several times daily. If more than two coffee enemas were performed in a single day or several were performed throughout the week, a second enema should be used. Use a tablespoon of cold pressed sunflower oil and a tablespoon of cold pressed flax seed oil mixed with enough water to fill the enema bag. These oils are very useful for ensuring cell wall integrity within the colon linings.

- Lemon – This is a good preventative enema. Squeeze the juice of ½ lemon into filtered warm water. Follow the instructions above.

4. Colonics:

- Colonics are more thorough than enemas. Enemas usually only reach the lower half of the large intestine whereas colonics are able to reach much deeper. I recommend colonics to all of my chronically ill patients. This is a very useful tool for colon detoxification and should be performed by an experienced colon therapist. A colon therapist should have a good knowledge of human anatomy with respect to the colon, utilize appropriate reflex points on the feet and trunk, and perform gentle massage techniques to assist in fecal removal. Finally, a good therapist will also understand the sensitivity of the ileocecal valve. This is the valve located between the small and large intestines. Following a colonic treatment, it is often necessary to manually close this valve by gently pressing on the right lower quadrant of the abdomen.

- Water is the main fluid used to irrigate the large intestine. I do not recommend forceful irrigation; gravity does just fine on its own.

- It may be necessary to undergo a series of treatments in order to overcome any impaction of fecal material that may likely be present. Home units are another alternative. However, it is best to receive treatments from a professional first before venturing on your own.

DO-IT-YOURSELF FORMULAS FOR THE COLON

If you want to save a good deal of money on supplements to make your bowels work properly; visit a whole foods market selling herbs. For about $50.00 you can have a one-year supply of digestive support! These formulas are both adapted from the book, *Curing with Cayenne and Its Herbal Partners*, by Sam Biser.

Herbal Laxative Formula:

This formula is designed for those with constipation or a slow bowel. Take one capsule after dinner. Continue increasing the dosage by one capsule each night until a bowel movement occurs every day. By volume combine, grind and put into capsules:

- 2 parts Aloe powder
- 3 parts Cascara Sagrada bark
- 1 part Oregon grape root
- 1 part Jamaican ginger root (increase if there is trouble digesting)
- 1 part Garlic bulb (increase if there is an infection)
- 1 part Habanero cayenne pepper (increase if there is any blood in the stool)

Constipation:

If the above formula looks to intimidating, purchase a bottle of magnesium from the health food store. Take two pills before bed on an empty stomach. The next night take three pills. Continue to increase the dosage until the following morning you have a noticeably loose bowel movement. Whatever the dosage was the night before (e.g. 5 pills) reduce the number by one pill and stay at that level. Only reduce in the future if you have loose bowel movements in the morning.

Irritable Bowel Formula:

For use with Crohn's disease, colitis, or any bowel problem where there is increased frequency. Take this formula 3 to 5 times per day beginning in the morning. Mix one heaping tablespoon in juice or water and drink. Follow this by drinking another 8 to 16 ounces of water.

- 2 parts flax seed
- 2 parts apple pectin
- 2 parts bentonite clay
- 2 parts slippery elm inner bark
- 1 part peppermint
- 1 part activated charcoal
- 7 parts psyllium husk

LIVER CLEANSING

The liver performs many vital functions. Cleaning blood by neutralizing toxic substances is one. Nearly 80% of the blood supply received by the liver comes from the intestines. That means that if the colon is clean, the blood going to the liver will be relatively clean as well. However, if the colon is toxic, the blood going to the liver will also be toxic. Therefore, the first step in liver detoxification is colon cleansing as described above. Next, do the following:

Supplements:

- Antioxidants (3 per day).
  - Purchase a combination product that contains SOD, Vitamins A, C, E and glutathione.
- L-Glutamine powder (1 level tablespoon in water, 3X per day).
- Fatty Acids (avoid corn and safflower oil).
  - Flax seed oil (2 capsules per day).
  - Sesame oil (2 capsules per day).
  - Olive oil on salads.
- Enzymes
  - From plants. Should contain lipase and protease. (1 with each meal, 1 between meals, and 2 before bed, for a total of 8 per day).

Liver and Gallbladder Flush

This is a powerful way to eliminate gallstones and cleanse the liver at the same time. After completing this procedure it is quite likely that you will see a few gallstones in your next bowel movement. Congratulations, you have successfully cleansed your gall bladder. If there are many gallstones, repeat this process in a week or two. <u>This procedure is not recommended for people under 25 years of age, those with very large gallstones (detected from an ultrasound), or if you have a history of gallbladder problems.</u>

1. For five days, drink as much fresh apple juice or apple cider as your appetite will permit in addition to regular meals and the liver supplements listed above.
2. Noon on the fifth day, you should eat a normal lunch.
3. 3 hours later, take two teaspoons of disodium phosphate (liquid phosphorous) dissolved in about one ounce of hot water with a squeeze of lemon (for taste).
4. 2 hours later, repeat step 3.
5. For your evening meal, you may have any freshly squeezed citrus juice and any citrus fruit.
6. Then at bedtime, you may do one of the following:
    a) ½ cup of unrefined olive oil followed by a small glass of grapefruit juice; or
    b) ½ cup of warmed unrefined olive oil blended with ½ cup of lemon juice; or
    c) 3 egg yolks mixed with ½ cup of cream.
7. Following step 6, you should go immediately to bed and lie on your right side with your right knee pulled up close to your chest. Stay in this position for 30 minutes.
8. The next morning, 1 hour before breakfast, take 2 teaspoons of disodium phosphate, dissolved in 2 ounces of hot water.

If you experience any nausea after drinking the olive oil, it should soon dissipate. Should vomiting occur, do not try to flush your gallbladder again until you have taken the liver supplements for 6 weeks.

KIDNEY CLEANSING

The kidneys are not only responsible for eliminating water-soluble waste products; they help regulate blood pressure as well. It is very important to keep these filters clean. The kidneys should be flushed periodically with the following formula:

- Juice of 1 lemon.
- Juice of ½ lime.
- 16 to 32 ounces of distilled water.
- A pinch of cayenne pepper.
- Maple syrup or honey to taste [optional].

Juniper Berry Tea
An alternate flush is a juniper berry tea. The juniper berries need to be very fresh and juicy. They have a soothing effect on the kidneys as well as anti-bacterial properties. Take one tablespoon of juniper berries with 20 ounces of water. Simmer for 15 minutes. Drink what remains 3-4 times throughout the day.

SKIN CLEANSING

Skin is the largest tissue of the body. One of its many functions is to detoxify the body. If you have ever experienced skin eruptions like acne, psoriasis or hives, chances are these blemishes were related to the detoxifying efforts of your body.

1) Brush your skin thoroughly with a loofah or other skin brush made from natural fibers. It is important to brush with a circular motion beginning at your feet and working your way toward the heart. This increases lymphatic drainage and circulation. Brush your abdomen in a circular motion from the lower right to the lower left. Women should not brush their breast tissue.

2) Rub your skin completely with a mixture of equal parts olive and cold pressed castor oil.

3) Immerse yourself in a hot bath for 15 minutes. Be careful, you are very slippery. The bath allows the oils to penetrate to the deepest levels of the skin.

4) After the bath, get under the covers, or put on several layers of clothes, and sweat for 1 hour.

5) Finally, take a shower to clean off.

You may follow this routine as much as you like. If you can't stand being greasy, then do step 1 each day followed by a hot bath with one cup of sea or Epsom salt added. Sweating is the key, so make sure your bath is hot. Of course, caution is needed with anyone who suffers from high blood pressure, dizziness or is sensitive to heat.

FASTING

To fast is to abstain from food for a chosen period of time. Fasting does two very important things. 1. It gives the body a rest from the energy-gulping job of digesting food. 2. It aggressively detoxifies the body.

Some people do what is called a juice fast, in which they eat no solid foods. Others abstain from both food and juice altogether, while drinking large amounts of water. Both are acceptable forms of fasting. The discipline and self-control required to fast, when done regularly, will translate into other areas of your life. Like most things, there are smart and not-so-smart ways to fast.

If you are only skipping a meal or two, you can get away with an abrupt start to a fast, but anything longer requires a little planning and preparation. I suggest doing a limited diet of vegetables and fruits with a few bites of lean meat for at least 3 days prior to any fast 1 day or longer. During those 3 preparation days, include some of the cleansing activities mentioned above in your routine. This will not only make the fast easier, but will greatly enhance its effects.

All of the side effects previously mentioned in the, *What Should I Expect* paragraph above are likely with a fast. The degree however, varies and is dependent upon the amount of toxins in your body and how well you have prepared for the fast.

Toxins in your body are like background noises. The more of them there are, the louder you have to talk in order to get your message across. Those experienced with fasting often relate how they feel "clear headed" and have finely tuned senses after a day or so of fasting. This is understandable, since you now have a lower toxic load. Begin slowly with the plan of increasing the amount of time you fast and you will see remarkable results as well.

Final Thoughts

Detoxification is perhaps the greatest need for the chronically ill. The lack of understanding by the medical community in general regarding even the most basic detoxification methods saddens me greatly. My chronically ill patients often tell me that their medical physician rarely discussed diet, rest, exercise and detoxification. If I was chronically ill and my doctor did not discuss or encourage a detoxification program, I would consider looking for someone else.

You do not have to do all of the programs mentioned above. Doing just one will help your body to function better. However, I strongly urge those who have suffered for a long time with any sort of illness, to use most or all of these programs on a regular basis. You will not regret it. Be sure to consult with someone knowledgeable in detoxification procedures before jumping right in. There are also many good resources available in the library, bookstore and on the Internet.

PREPARING FOODS

I have often seen patients who become sensitive to high quality foods. One of the reasons for this is that the foods are improperly prepared. Food preparation is one of the keys to eating healthy.

GRAINS, NUTS & SEEDS

The two easiest ways to increase the nutritional value of grains, nuts and seeds is through sprouting or soaking. There are enzymes within these foods that prevent them from sprouting. They also prevent the release of important nutrients. Usually all that is required to deactivate the enzymes is water. After learning the very simple techniques below, try the nuts and seeds in salads, sandwiches, vegetable dishes, as a breakfast cereal, and as additions to breads and baked goods. Sprouted grains should be eaten lightly steamed or added to soups or casseroles.

SPROUTING GRAINS & SEEDS

Use a mason jar with a screen insert. Fill the jar one third of the way with seeds or grains. Fill the remainder of the jar with filtered water and let stand overnight. The next morning, rinse the seeds well. Invert the jar and let it sit at an angle so that it can drain, and allow air to circulate. The seeds should be rinsed every few hours, or at least twice per day. In one to four days the sprouts will be ready. Rinse well. Remove excess moisture and place the now sealed jar in the refrigerator.

Almost any grain or seed can be sprouted. Flax and oat seeds however, are difficult. Also, it has been discovered that sprouted alfalfa can lead to chronic inflammatory conditions. One should avoid this sprout. Sprouts may be eaten regularly but not daily. They contain certain irritating substances that prevent animals from eating their roots. The old adage applies, "too much of anything can be bad".

SOAKING GRAINS & NUTS

Place the grains or nuts (beans should be soaked as well) in a large bowl. Add water and either a teaspoon of whey or a tablespoon of lemon juice. Make sure that the water level is 1/3 higher than the level of the grains. Place a clean towel or cheesecloth over the top of the bowl. Soak for 12-24 hours. This solution will soon become acidic. The acidic medium neutralizes phytates (mineral blocking agents) and begins the breakdown of carbohydrates, which allows you to obtain optimum nourishment from grains. It also provides lactic acid to the intestinal tract to facilitate mineral uptake. After 12-24 hours, drain the water, rinse thoroughly and prepare according to any recipe. You will notice a pleasant difference the next time you decide to make black bean soup - no socially unacceptable side effects.

GRAIN MILLS

Since our daughter Alyssa began eating solid foods my wife and I have been searching for the best foods we could find. As all parents know, kids love bread. However, we were displeased with the quality of bread sold in the stores. The few nutritionally acceptable breads we found cost between $3 and $5 per loaf. This adds up with a growing family. We were willing to purchase the more expensive breads, but even they are somewhat processed. This means that certain ingredients are either added (preservatives) or removed (oils and fiber). Our solution was to invest in a grain mill. This small, yet powerful devise crushes any hard grain into fine flour in just a few seconds. Since buying our mill we no longer buy bread in the store - we don't even want it. What a difference fresh ingredients make!

There are many machines on the market. We chose one called the Whisper Mill, which comes with a lifetime guarantee. It gets its name from the fact that it is several times quieter than its competitors. The good ones cost around $230. The investment may sound like a lot, but when you do the math, it pays for itself rather quickly. Additionally, you will find that the health and taste benefits far outweigh the cost.

The decision to purchase a grain mill comes with a few other requirements. Namely, you must buy and store grains. The grains themselves are very inexpensive. It is the shipping charges that can add up. Thankfully, there are distributors or co-ops in nearly every state. They put together a network of grain buyers, make a large order and then divide it up. As for storing grain, most types can sit in a sealed container for many years.

From start to finish, a loaf of the healthiest fresh bread can be made for about $0.50. There are many different ways to prepare bread. You can make a loaf in about 80 minutes with a simple bread machine, or make large batches of dough at one time. Dough can be tightly wrapped and frozen for future use. For those who are interested, I have put some numbers and websites in the resources section.

MILK

Milk is one of the most common food allergens I find in my practice. How the milk has been prepared and what has been added to it are two important reasons why. Also, allergies are more prevalent in people with genetic deficiencies, intestinal irritability or among those who consume large amounts of milk-based products.

The nutritional value and digestibility of milk has been limited by pasteurization - the process that prevents milk from spoiling by killing off the probiotics (native bacteria). It is true that spoiled milk can be a health problem, but so is drinking milk without any probiotics. Probiotics help digest the large proteins within milk, which are one of the prime irritants of the linings of the small intestine. The bacteria also acidify the milk which breaks down lactose – a substance many people cannot tolerate.

I do not recommend drinking milk to my patients. Instead, I suggest that they choose dairy products that have probiotics within them from culturing. Culturing is simply the process of adding certain bacteria back into the milk, thereby regaining some of the nutrients that were lost through processing. Sour cream, cottage cheese, yogurt and kefir are all cultured milk products. If you are interested in making your own cultured milk products, two of the easiest are piima or kefir.

Piima is a combination of five probiotics organisms that are lost during the pasteurization process. Kefir is easier to make than piima since it will grow in a wider temperature range. Kefir is an extremely beneficial beverage for children because of its immune boosting properties. It is also easy for most people with lactose intolerance to digest and may even be prescribed to candida suffers. Try adding kefir to any recipe that calls for milk. To make kefir or piima, you will need to purchase a "starter" from a distributor (see: RESOURCES). From the starter, you will be able to make a continuous supply of cultured dairy products.

HEALTH CABINET

Everyone should take responsibility for their health. This means having some understanding of how their body works and what it takes to keep it running smoothly. I therefore recommend that you have certain health supplies at home for prevention and recovery purposes. This chapter will help. This list is in no way exhaustive but is instead primarily designed for informational purposes.

Since you are a complex being, recipe style information would be insufficient for your needs. Before jumping in with both feet, you should combine this information with other health-related materials and the advice of your natural doctor. Do not waste your time asking a traditional doctor about supplements or herbs unless they use them in their office. They will be quick to try to discredit them. Despite the tremendous acceptance of natural healthcare methods among the general public in the last decade or so, there is still a significant amount of animosity between the competing healthcare systems. Even if you found a doctor who was open to natural ideas, unless he works with natural remedies every day, he will have little to offer. It would be like trying to get your email from the post office.

I have put in table format a few main topics and broken them down into sections with the vitamins or minerals listed as well as the herbs that promote health.

Herbs are immunoregulators. This means that they boost the immune system when it is suppressed and lower the immune system when it is working too well. I have included herbal recommendations for each of the main topics. If you want to try them, perhaps the easiest way is to make a tea. Teas are a good way to include health-building herbs into your daily life (see: Home Remedies, at the end of this chapter). The herbs can also be purchased from the health food store or bought online. They are safe for children, although I recommend buying tinctures already designed for children from Herbs For Kids, or Trilight Herbs (see: RESOURCES). These companies have already done the work for you by designing tinctures with condition specific herbs such as BactaMune for bacterial infections and ViraMune for viral infections. They have also used glycerin as the primary stabilizing medium, which has a sweet pleasant taste for kids. My children call it their, "good stuff."

When considering dosages, the manufacturer's recommendations are safe for any adult. However, I often use dosages 3 and 4 times the recommended level. I do not suggest this unless you have first discussed a protocol with your natural health doctor. Where I do make recommendations, they are for adults. To adjust the dosage for children calculate amounts by the child's weight compared to the weight of an adult of the same sex. Use 120 pounds for a female and 150 pounds for a male. In other words, a girl who weighs 60 pounds would take half the amount of an adult. A boy of 50 pounds would take one-third the amount of an adult.

BLOOD SUGAR SUPPORT

Blood sugar imbalances like hypoglycemia can result from a number of problems including eating too many carbohydrates and fatigued adrenal glands.

MINERALS	*Vanadium* *Chromium* These two are trace minerals that are needed in far smaller amounts than other more common minerals like calcium. They however, how powerful effects on blood sugar and are greatly missed by the body when not present in sufficient quantities.
HERBS	*Bilberry* *Fenugreek* *Bitter Melon* Used in combination, these herbs help with blood sugar handling problems by decreasing inflammation, normalizing hormonal functions, and acting as powerful antioxidants.
OTHERS	*Alpha Lipoic Acid* *B-Vitamins*

IMMUNE SYSTEM SUPPORT

Some sort of immune support should be taken on a regular basis. If you have a chronic condition (allergies, pain, infections) then the support should be daily.

VITAMINS	*Vitamins A and C* These are the nutrients which we use up rapidly when we are sick such as a cold or flu. Taking these hourly when sick is recommended. Vitamin C can be taken to bowel tolerance. This means that you should keep taking it until you have a very loose bowel movement. When this happens reduce your dosage. A and C combinations have also been useful in bladder infections (cystitis).
HERBS	*Echinacea* There are more than 400 studies demonstrating how this herb can benefit the immune system in various ways. Purchase or make a tincture with this herb as well as astragalus and/or licorice root *Others* Garlic and onions (eat raw or slightly cooked). Use liberally. Garlic has long been known as an infection fighter. Cayenne pepper can be ingested regularly to aid in blood cleansing, lung support and immune building. Start with just a pinch in water and work your way up to 1 teaspoon.
OTHERS	*Thymus Tissue* Those with chronic stress or chronic illnesses such as allergies or coughs will often require thymus tissue. The thymus gland is the center of the immune system. These can usually only be purchased from a healthcare provider.

ANTI-INFLAMMATORIES

Inflammation is a major part of every chronic illness. Therefore control and reduction is a key to health.

EFA's	*Black Currant Seed Oil (BCSO)* BCSO is often used in place of aspirin or acetaminophen. Aspirin and the other medications work by blocking the production of prostaglandin (PG) hormones. BCSO, on the other hand, works to bring imbalanced levels of PG back into balance. Certain headaches, muscle aches, hangovers, some menstrual symptoms and other inflammatory conditions can often be helped by BCSO. Try this instead of aspirin.
HERBS	*Turmeric* This herb is what gives curry its yellowish color. This herb is best taken as a pill or as a tincture. *Willow Bark (meadow sweet)* The original source of aspirin. 1 to 2 dropperfuls of tincture or 1 to 2 cups of tea.
OTHERS	*Manganese* Valuable in decreasing pain and speeding healing in sprains and fractures. A dose of six per day can be useful in aiding bone and ligament healing after the initial (acute) phase is over. *Proteolytic Enzymes* Taken on an empty stomach, enzymes can aid in the reduction of inflammation and the repair of damaged tissue.

ANTI-HISTAMINES

Useful in allergic reactions including food allergies, skin contact allergies, and some bug bites. In contact allergies and bug bites, natural anti-histamines are not as strong as over-the-counter anti-histamines. However, typical anti-histamine side effects such as drowsiness are usually not experienced.

MINERALS	*Calcium Lactate* When itchy skin, hives, muscle cramps or a sun burn occur, calcium lactate will help. Many women have achieved considerable relief from menstrual cramps by taking up to one Calcium Lactate every 15 minutes at the onset of cramps and one per hour after they begin to subside. It is usually used in conjunction with hydrochloric acid and essential fatty acids.
EFA's	*Vitamin F(essential fatty acids)* Essential fatty acids such as wheat germ oil, fish oil, and flax seed oil help calcium to get into our cells, especially in soft tissues like the skin, lips and tongue, and muscles. Vitamin D and vitamin F are exact opposites in respect to calcium. Many symptoms of too much sun are really symptoms of vitamin F deficiency and low cellular calcium. I have helped many women with hot flashes by suggesting a vitamin F product with iodine taken for at least three to four weeks.
HERBS	*Cloeus Forskoli* This herb helps to decrease the release of histamine from the mast cells and basophils, thereby decreasing inflammation and the allergic reaction. Others: chamomile, peppermint, ginger, and feverfew (make a tea with equal parts of these). Correcting allergic reactions often requires using anti-inflammatory herbs or vitamins as well. *Chlorophyll Ointment* A natural substance which can be applied topically to all sorts of skin problems especially burns. Chlorophyll ointment is extremely staining and will ruin anything it touches. If this is not an option, use aloe rather than chlorophyll. I recommend keeping an aloe vera plant growing around the house. Apply the fresh juice when needed.

OTHERS	*Hydrochloric acid (HCL)* Hydrochloric acid is normally made by the stomach and its supplementation is generally helpful for digestive conditions. However, since calcium is best absorbed in an acid medium, if calcium is low, adding HCL can be a benefit. Hydrochloric acid is available in products such as betaine hydrochloride or glutamic acid hydrochloride. Hydrochloric acid can be taken to help alleviate hay fever symptoms in many people. When hay fever symptoms flare up, take at least one tablet with each meal or as often as one tablet per hour as long as there is no burning in the stomach. If burning does occur, reduce the amount of HCL by one tablet.

MOOD SUPPORT

Depression, a common symptom of moodiness, is related to altered levels of a neurotransmitter called serotonin. Neurotransmitters are chemicals that stimulate specific receptors (neurons) in the brain producing a response. In the case of serotonin, when it stimulates its target receptors, a calming effect is produced which helps us to deal emotionally with the stresses of life.

VITAMINS	*Niacin, B6 and acetyl Co A* These are known to help in the production of serotonin, a mood enhancing compound in the brain. If these cofactors are low then the process will be inefficient at best and will likely result in low levels of serotonin.
OTHERS	*L-Tyrosine & 5-HTP* These work along the pathway that leads to the production of mood supporting compounds in the brain. One of these two will most likely be helpful.
HERBS	*St. John's Wort* *Lemon Balm Leaf* *Chamomile* *Passionflower* These herbs have long been known to help calm the mind and muscles. See: Stress Relief Tea below. *Others* Lavender essential oil. 1 to 3 drops in a hot bath.

LIVER SUPPORT (DETOXIFICATION)

The toxic environment we live in and the foods we eat make liver support a must. Detoxification is so important it has its own chapter.

AMINO ACIDS	*Cysteine* *Taurine* *MSM* These are sulfur containing substances. Five of the ten detoxification pathways in the liver require sulfur. Just be sure you do not have an allergy to sulfur before giving them a try.
HERBS	*Milk Thistle* This is a powerful but gentle detoxifier. It contains strong anti-oxidants called flavinoids that do a wonderful job protecting the liver. *Dandelion root* Use as a tea (add some honey for taste)

DIGESTIVE SUPPORT

"Heal the gut, fix the patient"

SUPPLEMENTS	*HCL* Hydrochloric acid is helpful for many patients with heartburn, which often results from low HCL production. It may also be helpful for those who eat and feel a heavy sensation in their stomach as if the food is not being digested. Stop taking if burning is experienced. *Plant enzymes* Aid in food digestion. *L-glutamine* A very good food source for the cells of the small intestine. It has anti-inflammatory properties. *Probiotics* Bacteria that is common in the intestines. These are often depleted in those with a poor diet or who have undergone recent courses of antibiotics. *Essential fatty acids* Powerful anti-inflammatory agents for the intestines.
HERBS	*Slippery Elm bark & Marshmallow root.* I use these to soothe the gut in cases where I suspect inflammation. *Others:* *Berberine* (anti-bacterial) *Artemicia* (anti-parasitic)

HOME REMEDIES

Here are two teas that can be very helpful. These recipes came from the book: Herbs for Health and Healing, by Kathi Keville.

Liver Tea

1 teaspoon of:

Dandelion Root
Milk Thistle Seeds

½ teaspoon of:

Licorice Root
Ginger Rhizome

1 quart of water

Combine the ingredients in a sauce pan and bring to a boil. Turn down heat and simmer for fifteen minutes. Strain and drink 1 cup a day. Add some honey for taste (optional). Try drinking this tea on a regular basis. Double or triple the batch and have it over ice throughout the week.

Cold and Flu Tea

½ teaspoon of:

Peppermint Leaves
Hyssop Leaves
Yarrow Leaves
Elder Flowers
Shizandra Berries

1 quart boiling water

Combine herbs and pour the boiling water over them. Let this mixture steep for 20 minutes. Strain and drink throughout the day (at least one cup every 1-2 hours). If you can't find the herbs, use a tincture with the same ingredients. Simply add ½ dropper full of the tincture to hot water and drink.

Here are a couple of other remedies I have used:

Cough Syrup
2 cups of honey
4 peeled and halved garlic cloves
½ peeled onion
2 tablespoons of marshmallow root
3 tablespoons water

Combine ingredients in an oven-safe container. Place in the oven at the lowest heat setting (approximately 150 degrees) for 3 hours. Strain and let cool. Store this mixture in the refrigerator. Take 1 tablespoon at a time. Great for kids with sore throats or dry coughs.

Stress Relief Tea
(A recipe from the Bulk Herb Store)

One part Passion Flower
One part Chamomile Flower
One part Oat Straw
One part Peppermint

Combine all of these ingredients together in a large, clean jar. To make one serving, take out one teaspoon at a time and add one cup of boiling water. Allow the tea to steep for 10 – 20 minutes. Strain and drink.

CARING FOR CHILDREN

If you want healthy children who can withstand disease including colds and ear infections, you must invest in their nutrition. From my experience and observation, around 80% of the vitality of children depends upon what they eat. The following guidelines, contained throughout this chapter, may be quite an adjustment for some parents to make, but they may represent the best gift you can provide for your children.

Organic foods make a big difference. Not only are they significantly higher in vitamin and mineral levels, they are also free from harmful chemicals. It is believed by many that the pesticides present in non-organic foods must not be harmful to the body since people do not get sick soon after eating them. However, small amounts of toxic material, ingested on a regular basis, will eventually accumulate in the body's tissues. Foods sprayed with pesticides or injected with antibiotics or hormones will contribute to the overall toxic load of the body, which may lead to the symptoms of toxicity. You will do your children a huge favor by offering them organic foods. For more information on the topic of toxins, see: SECTION III: Detoxification.

By helping children get good nutrients, you will increase their immune system's ability to fight off unwanted invaders and give them a good start in life, even before they are born.

BEFORE BIRTH

The development of a baby while in the mother's uterus is an amazing process with millions of chemical reactions taking place every minute. The birth of a healthy child is dependent upon this process receiving all the nutritional support required from the mother without her body removing anything from it. When the mother is not healthy she will not provide the essential nutrients for the child. In some cases, she may in fact take from the child in order to support her own tired tissues. For instance, a mother with fatigued adrenal glands will use the adrenal hormones produced for the child to support her own needs. This mother may feel better when pregnant than otherwise. However, stress is placed on the baby's adrenal glands. This usually results in infants who are cranky and cry all the time.

When a mother's nutrients are low, the child may be born with a compromised immune system, which leads to a life of increased sickness. A worse scenario occurs about two percent of the time in the general population, where a child is born with a malformation or birth defect.

In 1990, birth defects accounted for 21.5 percent of all infant deaths in the United States. They were broken down according to the systems they affected:

Heart - 32%
Respiratory - 14%
Nervous System - 13%
Chromosomal - 12%
Other - 29%

Compared to the general population, certain segments, such as women with insulin-dependent diabetes or those who have previously given birth to a child with neural tube defects, have an increased risk of delivering malformed babies.

A neural tube defect is a malformation of the brain or spinal cord during development. Spina bifida, where the spinal cord is exposed, and anencephaly, where most or all of the brain is missing are two common defects associated with the nervous system. These two neural tube defects occur each year in about 4,000 pregnancies. The Center for Disease Control (CDC) estimates that up to 3,000 of these birth defects could be prevented if women consumed folic acid before pregnancy and during early pregnancy.

A woman who wants to become pregnant and have a baby should take several steps to ensure that her body is healthy and able to support her child when the time comes. Here is my basic list:

- *Drink Water* – Most people are functionally dehydrated. Many symptoms people have such as fatigue and headaches can simply be the result of insufficient amounts of water. Water intake is also critical to proper detoxification.
- *Detoxify* – Our bodies store excess toxins. Removing these is a key piece to overall health and tissue function. If birth control pills have been part of a woman's life prior to becoming pregnant, I often recommend that she detoxify her body for at least one year. See: SECTION III: Detoxification.
- *Exercise* – Exercise is beneficial for every tissue in your body. It will help with labor and delivery by strengthening pelvic and leg muscles and increasing stamina. The lungs and all other organs will also be supported through exercise. See: SECTION III: Exercise.
- *Eat Healthy* – The only way to ensure that the proper nutrients your baby needs are present is to obtain them from your diet. Not only is eating the right foods important, but avoiding the wrong foods is also a key to keeping the nutrients you already have. See SECTION III: Diet.
- *Supplementation* – It makes good sense, in our increasingly toxic and stress filled world, to fortify your body with the nutritional vitamins and minerals that support daily function. For the pregnant woman and those women wanting to get pregnant, high quality

> nutritional supplementation is critical. My foundational recommendations include: a multivitamin designed for women, a multimineral, and essential fatty acids. In some cases, other specific supplements may be required depending upon the current and past health of the patient. More information is given throughout this chapter.

In the chapter, Diet I talk about listening to your body. This means paying attention to changes before and after you eat. The signs are the same for a pregnant or non-pregnant mother, with one exception. The child inside the pregnant mother will also provide some clues. If the mother eats a food that her body handles well but the baby does not, he may begin to move and kick in *excess* (kicking is a normal part of development). He may also hiccup. These are not good signs. A mother should take notice of these reactions and should avoid irritating foods in the future, thereby reducing the stress on the baby.

NEWBORNS

The single most important thing a mother can do for her newborn's future health is to breastfeed. Breast milk is perfectly designed for your baby's physical and mental development. Here are a few examples:

Immune system development:

- During the first few days of a baby's life, the mother's mammary glands will produce colostrum, an immune boosting substance, which helps protect against colds, flu, polio, staph infections and viruses.
- No matter how long the mother breast-feeds, antibodies from her milk are supplied to the baby, and act as a continual immune system builder.
- Breast milk is a powerful anti-biotic. So much so, that a few drops administered directly into the ear canal can be used effectively for the treatment of childhood ear infections.

Mental development:

- Higher performance IQ scores.
- Improved long-term brain function.
- Higher verbal IQ scores.

As a general rule, breast-fed babies tend to be more robust and more intelligent. They are also less likely to suffer from allergies and intestinal difficulties than those on formula. They may not be as fat though. Comparing breastfed and bottle-fed children, you will probably notice that the bottle-fed children are more plump. This is just my observation. I do not have any research to back this up. For fun, take a look for yourself.

BREAST MILK QUALITY

It must be emphasized that all breast milk is not the same. The quality of mother's milk depends greatly on her diet and overall health. If a mother regularly eats poor quality foods such as fast foods and processed foods, she should not expect her milk to provide as many benefits as milk from the mother who makes wiser dietary choices.

Despite what some pediatricians say, pesticides and other toxins will be present in mother's milk if they are present in the diet. All care should be taken to consume organic foods of both plant and animal origin during pregnancy and lactation. Breast milk contains a great deal of fat. Eating organic foods provides more of the important omega-3 fatty acids needed for baby's optimal development. Hydrogenated fats should be strictly avoided – they are poisons (see: SECTION III: Diet & Foods). They will accumulate, leading to reduced quality milk and potential problems for the infant. Stress also plays a role in overall breast milk quality. The less stress on mom, the greater the milk supply and the greater the breast milk quality.

Supplements for Mom

To ensure that developing children receive their required nutrients, it is a good idea for mothers to use supplements while they are pregnant and as they breastfeed. Supplements however, are not enough. Scientists know only a minuscule amount pertaining to the substances in our food. Widely recognized vitamins and minerals are only a small piece of the dietary puzzle. Vital nutrients are discovered each year, which are not present in most supplements. Supplements can have their own share of problems as well. The label may tell you what is in the bottle, but it says nothing about the type (natural or synthetic), quality, or the degree to which the pills have been processed. Therefore, an above average diet becomes essential. I often tell mothers to concentrate on eating whole, unprocessed foods to ensure that their baby is getting the essential nutrients it has been designed to utilize.

Please refer to Section III: Diet & Foods for detailed dietary guidelines. For now, the lactating mother should make sure that she receives plenty of:

- *Water* – by far the easiest thing a nursing mother can do to help herself and her milk supply, is to drink plenty of water. ½ - 1 gallon per day is not too much.
- *Eggs, liver, chicken, fish and other animal proteins* - These ensure that her milk will have proper amounts of vitamin B12, A and D, as well as all-important minerals like zinc.
- *Cod liver, fish or flax seed oil.*
- *Stock made from bones.*
- *Whole milk products* - Pasteurized milk is acceptable if it is not homogenized and should be cultured with Kefir grains for 12 hours. See instructions on culturing grains in the chapter, Preparing Foods. The right dairy products will add size to your baby. Our first two daughters, Alyssa and Audra, weighed 6 lbs. 12 oz. and 6 lbs. 6 oz. respectively. Our third daughter, Brooke, weighed 8 lbs. 6 oz. (2 lbs. heavier!) Brooke's delivery was also the easiest by far. Alyssa - Cesarean section; Audra - Born at home after 30 hours of labor, 11 hours of hard labor and 2 hours of pushing; Brooke – Born at home after 12 hours of labor, 3 hours of hard labor and 2 minutes of pushing. The only dietary difference was a conscious effort on my wife's part to eat more wholesome dairy products.

FORMULAS

Breast-feeding should ideally be continued for at least six months to a year or more. If a mother is unable to breast-feed, or if her milk is not of good quality due to poor nutrition, a homemade baby formula can be used. I encourage the mother wanting to make her own formula to purchase the book <u>Nourishing Traditions</u>, by Sally Fallon.

Store-Bought Formulas

Do everything you can to avoid commercial formulas. These products are highly processed and contain many chemical preservatives and carcinogens (cancer causing agents). According to Sally's book, "Milk-based formulas often cause allergies while soy-based formulas contain mineral-blocking phytic acid, growth inhibitors and plant forms of estrogen compounds that can have adverse effects on the hormonal development in the infant. Soy-based formulas are also devoid of cholesterol, needed for the development of the brain and nervous system."

If store bought formulas are your only option, you can purchase a formula from the health food store that is rice-based and organically grown. In addition, to avoid any colicky episodes, you will probably need to supplement your child with ½ capsule of plant enzymes and ¼ capsule of probiotics (natural bacteria) per bottle of formula. Also, grated liver can be added to this formula as well. We did this with Alyssa, our first daughter, before we knew about Sally's formulas. She turned out to be very healthy. But remember, we did everything else in this section too!

DIETARY GUIDELINES FOR CHILDREN

When the mother is ready to stop breast feeding or would like to incorporate other foods into the child's diet, here is what I suggest:

Baby's First Foods

Baby's earliest solid foods should be animal foods. The digestive system of a baby, although immature, is better equipped to supply enzymes for breaking down fats and proteins, rather than carbohydrates. Therefore, a wise supplement for all babies—whether breast-fed or bottle fed, is a slightly undercooked organic egg yolk per day, beginning at around five months.

Make sure that the egg yolk is not overcooked. Boil the eggs for only 3 ½ minutes. The yolk will come out soft and the middle will be warm. You may also cook the egg over-easy and give the runny yolk to your child. This approach is a little messier. Overcooking the yolk destroys the enzymes and makes digestion more difficult. If your baby experiences digestive complaints such as gas after eating an egg yolk, then it is probably overcooked.

Egg yolk supplies many substances needed for mental and nervous system development including cholesterol, essential amino acids and omega-3 long-chain fatty acids. These fatty acids are essential for the development of the brain. The white part of the egg, which contains difficult-to-digest proteins, should not be given before the age of one year. Also, small amounts of grated, raw organic liver may be added occasionally to the egg yolk after six months. Liver is rich in iron, the one mineral that tends to be low in mother's milk.

Carbohydrates in the form of fresh, mashed bananas or apples can be added after the age of six months. These fruits are rich in amylase enzymes and are easily digested by most infants; there are exceptions. Most babies do very well with bananas. Ours however, did not. Little Alyssa would develop a small rash on her face as well as a bad attitude. Remember that all children are created with their own special needs.

Ten Months

At the age of about ten months, meats, other fruits and vegetables may be introduced, one at a time so that any adverse reactions may be observed. Soups are perhaps the easiest way to go. You can make a large pot of soup and use it as your baby food. Use meat stock to ensure the presence of beneficial fats and add vegetables. It is usually easiest to purée the soup. Once several teeth appear, leave the soup a little chunky so that baby can learn to chew. It is also advisable to begin feeding your baby small amounts, a tablespoon or two, of buttermilk, yogurt or Kefir (a fermented milk beverage). Of course these should all be organic foods. These substances contain beneficial bacteria that aid in digestive health.

One Year

In our society it is common to feed babies cereal grains as a first food. Babies however, are not fully equipped to handle cereals, especially wheat, before the age of one year because they produce only small amounts of amylase - an enzyme needed for the digestion of grains. The most common carbohydrate enzyme in the small intestine of a baby is lactase. This enzyme helps with the digestion of milk. Because the enzymes needed for digesting grains are present in only small numbers, many doctors have warned that feeding cereal grains too early can lead to grain allergies later on. Some experts prohibit all grains before the age of two. This is not necessary if the grains are properly prepared.

Preparing Grains

Proper grain preparation produces high levels of nutrients and aids in digestion. See: SECTION III: Preparing Foods.

Other Considerations

A baby's immature liver may have difficulty converting carotenoids to vitamin A, so be careful with orange vegetables. If your baby's skin develops a yellowish color, discontinue orange vegetables for a time. Above all, do not deprive your baby of animal fats - he needs them for optimum physical growth and mental development. Mother's milk contains over 50% of its calories as fat, much of it saturated fat, and children need these kinds of fats throughout their growing years.

Beyond One Year

Finally, once your baby is able to eat most foods, feed him the following:

- Eggs - omelets with veggies, soft boiled or over-easy eggs.
- Soups - homemade or organic store bought, made with all natural ingredients.
- Meats - turkey, chicken, occasionally roast beef and liverwurst (preferably from a Kosher deli).
- Fish - Cod, salmon or other cold water fish.
- Homemade Bread – The most nutritious bread that can be made is from grains ground at home. I discuss this topic in the chapter, The Maintenance Diet.
- Ezekiel Bread – this is a good alternative to homemade bread. This bread is a complete food made of seven or so sprouted grains. It may be purchased at most health food stores (Look in the freezer section).
- Green Veggies – spinach, green beans, peas and broccoli.
- Other Veggies – squash, cooked carrots, cooked onions, garlic
- Stews (a good way to add extra veggies to the diet)
- Fruit – kiwi, pears, plums, avocado and grapes.
- Grains – prepared (soaked) brown rice, spelt flour, and millet
- Oatmeal or Oat bran – easy to digest and easy to make. Try adding some real maple syrup and some Kefir. Your kids will ask for it just like Alyssa, "Obree, Obree, Obree".

Foods to Minimize

- Any inorganic food (veggies, fruit, meat).
- Citrus.
- Refined white flour - cakes, cookies, breads, crackers.
- White potatoes.
- Non-organic diary.

Foods to Avoid

Keep your baby away from processed junk foods as long as possible—but do not think that you can do this indefinitely. Unless you lock your child in a closet—or live in a closed community of like-minded parents—he will come in contact with junk foods sooner or later. His best protection is the optimal diet that you have given him during his infancy and your loving example and training in later years.

- Sodas, processed fruit drinks.
- Prepared and/or boxed foods.
- Most snacks.
- Fried foods
- Sugar and White Flour

These last two are ubiquitous, heavily refined foods in our society. Many "experts" say that sugar and flour are simply carbohydrates - an easy fuel source for the body. This is true. However, the form in which we eat sugar and flour is nowhere near their natural state. When examined naturally, carbohydrates are combined with vitamins, minerals, enzymes, protein, fat and fiber - the bodybuilding and digestion-regulating components of foods. In whole form, sugars and starches support life; but refined carbohydrates destroy life because they evaporate the body's nutrient reserves. When B vitamins are absent, for example, the breakdown of carbohydrates cannot take place, yet most B vitamins are removed during the refining process.

As the consumption of sugar has increased, so have all of the "civilized" diseases. According to Sally Fallon, author of the book, Nourishing Traditions, "Today, the average intake of sugar per year is around 170 pounds per person. Another large portion of all calories comes from white flour and refined vegetable oils. This means that over half of the diet must provide all of the nutrients to a body that is already under constant stress from its intake of sugar, white flour, and rancid and hydrogenated vegetable oils." Here is a list of the diseases directly related to refined food consumption:

- Anorexia
- Arteriosclerosis
- Atrophy of the pancreas
- Bone loss
- Candida overgrowth
- Dental decay
- Diabetes
- Elevated triglycerides
- Heart Disease
- High Cholesterol
- Hyperactivity
- Hypertrophy of the adrenal glands
- Hypertrophy of the liver
- Kidney Disease
- Liver disease
- Loss of concentration
- Shortened life span
- Skin degeneration

The above list is an abbreviated version of what sugar can do. Currently in our office we have photocopies of an article entitled, *59 Reasons to Avoid Sugar*. Each of these reasons comes directly from a peer-reviewed medical journal or similar reference. Do your very best to stay away from refined sugar.

Snacking

Snack time is important. I believe that parents inadvertently wreck their child's diet at snack time. Often, they are lured into believing that snack foods with vitamins are healthy. Kool Aid® and Fruit Rollups® will never be healthy no matter how much fruit juice or how many synthetic vitamins have been added. When I look in the typical parent's pantry, I find large amounts of potentially sickness causing snacks. The freezer is no better. Ice cream, popsicles, and waffles are commonplace. These things are not going to kill the child when eaten once in a while, but a closer look reveals that snack and junk foods are eaten with regularity. Think for a moment about your child's diet and see if they have gone even one day without some form of junk food. Most people haven't. Unfortunately, junk and snack foods have become the bribing tools of choice; rewards for good behavior. Space does not permit delving into this subject. Suffice it to say, snack foods are bad for reasons beyond nutrition alone. Do your best to limit junk snacks to times of celebration such as birthday parties and social gatherings.

What to Drink

Parents often give their kids fruit or flavored juices. These are often not good choices because they only provide simple carbohydrates and frequently spoil an infant's appetite for more nutritious foods. They are also processed and have no enzymes left, making them much harder to digest. Store bought apple juice, for instance, contains Sorbitol, a sugar-alcohol. Studies have linked failure to thrive in children with diets high in apple juice. High-fructose foods, like fruit juices and sodas are especially dangerous for growing children. If you have to buy store bought juice – definitely add powdered vitamin C (500mg). Store bought organic juices will often contain mold and pasteurized non-organic juices are full of sugar, which suppresses the immune system for up to 4 hours after ingestion. Vitamin C powder is a simple, inexpensive way to enhance the quality of store bought juices.

Water and Juices

Water is an essential food for your child once they stop breast-feeding. You will probably have a hard time getting your child to drink water if they have been drinking juice for any length of time. This demonstrates how powerful the desire for sugar can be. If you can't get your child to drink plain water, then add a small amount of juice. Gradually add less and less juice until they drink the real thing. Besides water, my wife and I have discovered the wonderful world of juicing. Freshly made vegetable and fruit juice is one of the best preventative measures you can give your child. It is full of live enzymes and body building nutrients that children need. Citrus juice, however, even freshly made, should only be given in small amounts, preferably diluted or mixed with other juices. When you decide to start juicing for your child's health, begin with the following:

- 3 carrots
- ½ apple

Your child will enjoy this sweet flavor. Don't be surprised if they ask for it regularly. Later, try adding some spinach (around 10 leaves or so), and a squeezed quarter of a lemon. Eventually, you will want to always include green vegetables. Juices can be the best way to add green leafy vegetables to the finicky child's diet, especially when they are combined in a base of carrot and apple juice.

When children are sick you should also include immune strengthening and bug killing foods in their juice like garlic and ginger. Just use a little bit at first. The taste is quite strong but the benefit is almost immediate. Here is a health building concoction we gave to our daughter during one of her green mucous episodes:

- 3 carrots
- ½ apple
- 10 spinach leaves
- 1 clove garlic
- 1 teaspoon ginger root
- Parsley
- ¼ lemon

It is hard to believe, but our daughter gobbled up this strong tasting drink. Again, parents will have a hard time getting their kids to drink these odd tasting juices if they have been raised on beverages high in sugar.

Sample Menu
This was a typical day for our first daughter when she was 18 months old:

Breakfast
- 1 to 2 eggs with 1 slice of Ezekiel bread (usually sesame seed); or,
- 1 ½ cup oat bran with added Kefir and/or real maple syrup; or,
- Leftover meat from dinner
- 4-6 oz of vegetable or fruit juice (freshly juiced)
- Fresh fruit

Snack

- Dried organic fruit (without any preservatives like sulfites) Apricots, dates, raisins; or,
- Small portion of graham crackers (made without partially hydrogenated oils) This is not a staple for us, but is a treat for her; or,
- ½ cup yogurt, plain with added berries; or,
- 1 cup Kefir, made into a shake with berries and stevia, an herb 30X sweeter than sugar.

Lunch

- Turkey or almond butter with jelly, or avocado sandwich on Ezekiel bread.
- Fruit or cooked veggie.

Dinner

- Broiled fish, baked chicken or organic turkey.
- A green veggie.
- Water or fresh juice.

It is okay to use butter, just buy organic. Sometimes this is the only way to get a child to eat broccoli!

COMMON PROBLEMS WITH KIDS

COLIC

The definition of colic is irritability and crying usually in the late afternoon or evening for three to six hours per day, three to six days per week, for three weeks to six months per year. I remember my grandmother telling me that she would frequently go to the pediatrician's office where she would be sent to a special room downstairs to let my mother cry until finally falling asleep. This episode was the main reason why my mother was an only child. There are several potential reasons why a baby has colic. Thankfully, there are natural therapies that can be extremely helpful for each cause.

Structural Causes

- *Birth trauma* – The use of forceps or vacuum suction often distorts the cranial bones to such an extent that their natural influences over the nerves that affect digestion are disrupted. Simple cranial corrections many times have a profound positive effect. When unnatural methods are not used to deliver a baby, he may still be in need of corrections in the lower spine and the cranium.
- *Car seats* - Make sure that the padding in the back of your baby's car seat goes all the way down past their buttocks. Sometimes the padding stops above the buttock region creating a drop-off, which places the baby in a slumped position. Both the drop-off and the poor posture place stress on the lowest vertebrae in the spine – the ones with direct nerve influence over digestion.

Digestive Causes

- *Food sensitivities* – In my opinion this is the most common cause of colic. Babies with colic regularly have gas and hike their knees up into their chest for relief. This clearly indicates improper digestion of some food. No mater what you have heard, the baby receives in breast milk whatever is eaten by the mother. The baby may be sensitive to a food that the mother has no reaction to whatsoever. Even the most seemingly benign food should be evaluated. I do this with applied kinesiology methods while testing with different food samples. If the baby is experiencing reflux as well, he should be put to sleep with one end of the bed elevated (a phone book under the mattress works well) and his head on the highest end. This helps to keep the food down in the stomach.

- *Microorganism infections* – Often mothers with fungal overgrowth will pass this problem on to their children. When present, food allergies will soon result, due to the disruption of the normal ecology of the intestines.

Environmental Causes

- *Over stimulation* – In some instances a baby is held too much or is exposed to too many bright lights and loud sounds. These stimuli are excitatory and lead to disrupted sleep, poor nursing and upset stomachs. Too little stimulation, such as a completely quiet environment is not healthy either. Place the child in an environment that has regular, but not excessive amounts of stimuli.

- *Hungry baby* – Some babies do not receive the full nourishment they require even if they are breastfed. Yes, breast milk is a perfect food, but only if all of it is consumed. The first portion of breast milk is lower in fat than the hind portion. The hind portion is the cream of the milk. When consumed the baby will be satiated and tend to sleep longer without waking up. The cream is also a soother of the intestines. If a baby nurses frequently but only for a short time, all he will be receiving will be the watery first portion and not the creamy hind portion. This baby will tend to be fussy and cranky. To make sure that the baby drains the entire breast stretch the time between feedings. He will eat well when he is hungry enough.

EAR INFECTIONS

Ear infections in a child are usually very painful and are often associated with crying, moodiness and tugging at the affected ear.

A fever may also be present. Children tend to have ear infections because the tube running between the back of the throat and the ears (Eustachian tube) is more horizontally aligned than an adult's, which is more vertical. If the Eustachian tube is not draining properly, fluid will accumulate and allow for the cultivation of microorganisms. As the microorganisms reproduce they increase the pressure inside the tube which is painful for the child.

Mucous producing foods such as dairy products and sugars are one of the reasons for poor Eustachian tube drainage. Food allergies are another source of mucous production and inflammation. If the child exclusively craves a certain food, they are often allergic to it.

If the infection is bacterial, antibiotics may help. However, repeated courses of antibiotics will promote the overgrowth of fungus in the gut leading to other health problems. Also, the infection may not be bacterial, but fungal in origin, in which case antibiotics will only create more problems.

A parent must differentiate between an ear infection and teething, which may cause jaw pain and muscle tension around the jaw so that the child pulls on their ears. When a true ear infection is present, correcting the uppermost bones of the neck and the bones of the cranium can be beneficial. The misaligned bones place tension on the muscle near the ear and restrict the openings of the Eustachian tube. Also, the child should be well hydrated and kept from sugary foods, refined white flour and dairy products. Finally, they should be checked for food allergies and microorganism infections.

VACCINATIONS

There are some topics in life that immediately evoke an emotional response no matter which side of the issue you are on. Whether or not to vaccinate your newborn child is one of them. Because so much emotion is involved, the prudent parent will seek credible information from both sides before making their decision.

For the record, I have three children less than four years of age. After looking into the topic for myself and evaluating the pros and the cons, none of them have been vaccinated. This does not mean that I believe that all children should not be vaccinated. Read the information below (and lots of other material) before making your decision.

There is a great deal of pressure from many sources to vaccinate your children. All sorts of guilt and condemnation await those parents who choose to do otherwise.

The U.S. has one of the highest vaccination rates in the world. If you follow the recommendations set up by the Centers for Disease Control and the American Academy of Pediatrics, your child will receive nearly 34 doses of ten different vaccines by the time they enter kindergarten.

What are the long-term effects on the human body? Several childhood conditions are escalating in this country such as asthma and attention deficit disorder. Many of us in the natural health field suspect a relationship between this conditions and vaccinations. Unfortunately, very few studies are underway to confirm or deny this suspicion.

Vaccination rates are increasing. American children born in 1948 were only required by state health officials to show proof of smallpox vaccination to enter school. For the American child born in 1998, getting in school requires being injected with 33 or 34 doses of 9 or 10 different viral and bacterial vaccines. Today, there are more than 200 vaccines being created by federal health agencies and drug companies, including Hepatitis C, D and E; Herpes simplex types 1 and 2; gonorrhea; rotavirus (diarrhea); Group A and B streptococcus; meningitis A, B and C; and HIV for AIDS. I am scared to think what the child born in 2008 will be required to undergo.

WHY I DIDN'T VACCINATE

Without question vaccinations have been a powerful force in the prevention of disease. However, in my opinion, in the U.S. today they are an abused form of health care. Below I have provided the five reasons why I chose not to vaccinate my three girls.

Toxic

- *Vaccinations shots are filled with toxic ingredients* – Genetic material from other infected animals, preservatives (formaldehyde and acetone, and heavy metals), antibiotics, and other chemicals are all injected into the closed system of the blood stream.
- *The blood stream* – most diseases for which children are vaccinated come from the air. The body has special defense systems to help fight these organisms if they are breathed into the nasal passages and lungs. However, when injected into the blood stream, these defenses are bypassed, which creates an immune response different than what was intended. In other words, vaccinations are a direct assault on the most guarded and protected system of the body.
- Vaccines are grown on animals such as chickens, monkey kidney cells, human fetal tissue (chicken pox vaccine) and infected tissues.
- *Thimerosal* – an organic form of mercury that is fifty times more potent than mercury. When an infant receives a vaccination shot containing thimerosal, they are actually receiving a dose of mercury 70 – 200 times higher than the recommended safe levels. Thankfully, the United States is reducing this ingredient in many vaccines…but not all.

Temporary

- Vaccinating your child does not guarantee that they will not contract the disease for which they were vaccinated. Some children get the disease as a result of being vaccinated. For example, the antibodies for Hepatitis B are not detectable in 30% and 50% of persons after 7 years despite having three doses of the vaccine. If immunity only lasts 7 years, babies vaccinated with hepatitis B vaccine may be candidates for more shots (boosters) at age seven (see more on Hepatitis B below).
- The only way you get permanent immunity is by getting the disease.

Type

- Most of the vaccinations given today are for non-life threatening diseases. Chicken pox for instance, is merely a nuisance. Once a child endures this condition he will have lifetime immunity. Others, like polio, are essentially non-existent in the United States. Then there are the vaccinations that make no sense whatsoever (except perhaps economically). Take Hepatitis B for example.

- *Hepatitis B* – People at high risk for getting Hepatitis B disease (which is transmitted by coming into direct contact with an infected person's body fluids) are IV drug users, prostitutes, prisoners, sexually promiscuous persons and babies born to infected mothers. Since this is true, why do most hospitals inject a Hepatitis B vaccine into babies before they even leave the hospital? I have yet to hear a reasonable explanation for this one.

  Hepatitis B is not life threatening. 90-95% of all hepatitis B cases recover completely after 3 to 4 weeks. Symptoms include: nausea, fatigue, headache, arthritis, jaundice and a tender liver. Interestingly, up to 17 percent of all hepatitis B vaccinations are followed by reports of fatigue and weakness, headache, arthritis and fever of more than 100 F.

Timing

- The vaccination schedule requires most babies to be fully vaccinated by the time they are two years old. This was the strongest reason why my children were not vaccinated. In my practice I see what simple foods can do to the health of a sensitive adult. It makes no sense to me then, given my experience and what I have already explained above, why a child with an underdeveloped immune system should be subject to such an extremely toxic substance at so young an age (some shots are given soon after they are born). The immune system of the child is dependent upon receiving support from the mother's breast milk, which contains certain antibodies that help prevent infection. Since breast feeding should last at least one year, it is possible that the child's immune system takes this long to fully develop.

- In Japan, the rate of Sudden Infant Death Syndrome (SIDS) almost disappeared when the vaccination program was stopped until after 2 years of age.

Tragedy

- As with any medical procedure, there are risks associated with vaccinations. The Food and Drug Administration established the Vaccine Adverse Events Reporting System (VAERS). Every year 12,000 to 14,000 hospitalizations, injuries, and deaths following vaccination are reported to VAERS. Experts suspect that numbers are much higher because not all parents report adverse reactions.
- A child who has had a previous severe reaction to a vaccination can be especially at risk for even more severe reactions if more vaccine is given.
- Monitor your child closely after vaccination. Call your doctor if you suspect a reaction. If your doctor is not concerned and you are, take your child to an emergency room.
- If your child is left permanently brain damaged or dies as a result of a vaccine reaction, you may be entitled to benefits under the National Childhood Vaccine Injury Act of 1986. By fall 1995, the federal vaccine injury compensation program had compensated nearly 1000 families at a cost of $600 million.

Obtain a copy of your state mandatory vaccination laws. Become educated about state vaccine requirements, your rights and legal exemptions to vaccination. In most states a religious exemption is permitted. Thankfully, in Colorado, parents are permitted to deny vaccinations for philosophical reasons as well.

WHEN I WOULD VACCINATE

Despite my strong views as outlined above, I would vaccinate my children under certain conditions.

- *When their immune systems are strong* - This usually means waiting until the age of 3 or 4. I would consider changing my mind on this point if there were an outbreak of a highly contagious life-threatening disease and a safe vaccine was available. However, in the U.S. that is not presently the case.
- *If I could not properly care for my child* – I am at a tremendous advantage. Since I work in the health field I am familiar with the subtle signs and symptoms of oncoming sickness. I am also able to support their immune systems with many of the remedies and recommendations provided in this book. I do not permit the weakening of their immune systems through prolonged lack of sleep, too many stimulating activities (television, video games etc.) or constant junk food indulgences. As a result, they are much healthier than many children their own age.
- *If my child were at significant risk to contract a disease that was life threatening or life altering.*
- *Traveling to a foreign country where there is a known abundance of a particular disease.*

For more information on this immensely important topic presented in a balanced format please see:

The National Vaccine Information Center
800-909-SHOT
www.909shot.com

TREATING SICK KIDS

There are many things that can be done to stimulate the immune system of a child who is starting to get sick. If your child begins acting out of sorts or has been exposed to sick children, do the following:

- Avoid all white bread products.
- Maximize vegetables, soups, vitamin C, and homemade juice drinks.
- No snack foods, sweets or store bought juices!
- If vomiting is a problem, do the best you can to give your child fresh made juices of apple, carrot, green vegetables, and especially garlic. This juice is far better than Gatorade, because it is full of enzymes that the body will use to dispose of the unwanted invader(s). Even if your child vomits up the juice, it only takes seconds for the intestinal track to absorb many of the beneficial nutrients. Try giving them just a small amount from a dropper if they can't ingest an entire cup worth.
- The other soothing beverage for sick children is warm organic chicken broth, sold in the health food store, which can be given in a sippy cup.
- Finally, take your child to the chiropractor for an adjustment of their upper neck and cranial bones; it will help their body rebound quickly.

FOOD REACTIONS

Pay close attention to the behavior of your child after eating certain foods. Junk foods often have immediate and dramatic effects on the behavior of children. Also, take a good look at your child's skin every day. Skin is one of the areas on the body that will let you know if something is not right. My wife frequently shows me new bumps or mild rashes that our girls develop after eating junk foods. These bumps are very tiny and are commonly found on the face and cheeks, although they may be anywhere. Look closely; you will certainly notice changes. When you do, tighten the reigns on your child's diet; or else, sickness may be just around the corner.

Doing all the right things does not mean your children won't get sick. Some sickness is good because it builds immunity. Chronic sickness, the type that we want to avoid, means that something is wrong.

Our girls have had their share of colds. However, not like other kids. At the time of this writing, our daughters are 4 years, 2 years and 7 months old. Since being born, Alyssa and Audra have been sick (with green mucous) a few times each. Alyssa has vomited once over a 24 hour period due to food poisoning from bad frozen vegetables. Our youngest, Brooke contracted a respiratory virus common in the Denver area at the age of two weeks and was put on a home nebulizer for three days. Besides this, she seems to be our healthiest baby. All of our girls are regularly around other children and are exposed to many different atmospheres, not to mention that I spend all day with sick people and bring their germs home with me. They have never had an ear infection, or been on antibiotics. I say this only to emphasize that it is possible to have a child with a strong immune system; one who is able to overcome illnesses and who is not always sick or on antibiotics. There is help and there is hope. A good diet is a must for a strong healthy child and regular chiropractic adjustments will help greatly.

SUPPLEMENTS
The right supplements can be very helpful for children. Getting them to take them is another problem. I have a hard enough time getting my adult patients to do it. Try hiding them in applesauce or soups. Whatever you do, do not give them their supplements with junk food. I have had this self-defeating behavior happen before. Here are a few supplements that should be around the home of all parents:

- Probiotics – ex. Lactobacillus acidophilus. These are friendly bacteria that can be purchased at any health food store. They are also found in high levels in cultured milk. These should be given with any form of sickness. 60 -70%

of our immune system resides in the linings of the gut. When you give these supplements you keep the gut healthy and strengthen the immune system at the same time.

- Immuplex – Or similar immune supporting supplement. These supplements contain spleen, thymus and other organ tissues that greatly enhance immune system function. They usually come in tablet form and will need to be crushed for the little ones.
- L-Glutamine – This is the primary food source for the cells in our small intestine and is given for the same reason as the Probiotics.
- Vitamin C powder – This is a must. If your child is not feeling well, has a bad attitude, or a food reaction, this supplement can be used. Start with around 500mg in homemade fruit juice. You may increase the dosage until your child has diarrhea. If this happens, simply cut back their dosage.

For more information on supplements are herbs see: SECTION III: Health Cabinet.

NEURO-IMMUNE TREATMENT (NIT)

Here is the abbreviated version of NIT that I discuss in SECTION III: Self Treatment.

There are many ways to desensitize the body, making it easier to overcome low grade infections and food sensitivities. This one is perhaps the easiest to perform and the one I recommend to parents. All you need to do is obtain a sample of body fluid. If your child has a runny nose, use the mucous. For a sore throat use some saliva. For digestive problems use a small amount of stool. Wrap up the appropriate fluid in some toilet or tissue paper. Only a small amount is required, about the size of a quarter is sufficient. You may put the sample in a plastic bag if desired. Next, hold this tissue against the chest of the child while you vigorously rub each of the areas below for 20 to 30 seconds. Be sure not to rub so that it hurts. Instead the pressure should be in the tickle range. That's it.

It is believed that this technique works by triggering the higher centers of the brain, resulting in a greater immune system response. When you externally expose your child to whatever bug is causing sickness and then treat the areas indicated below by rubbing, you will help the body overcome the infection. Try it and see. You will be amazed at the speed of recovery when this simple technique is performed, but don't forget to do everything else discussed above as well.

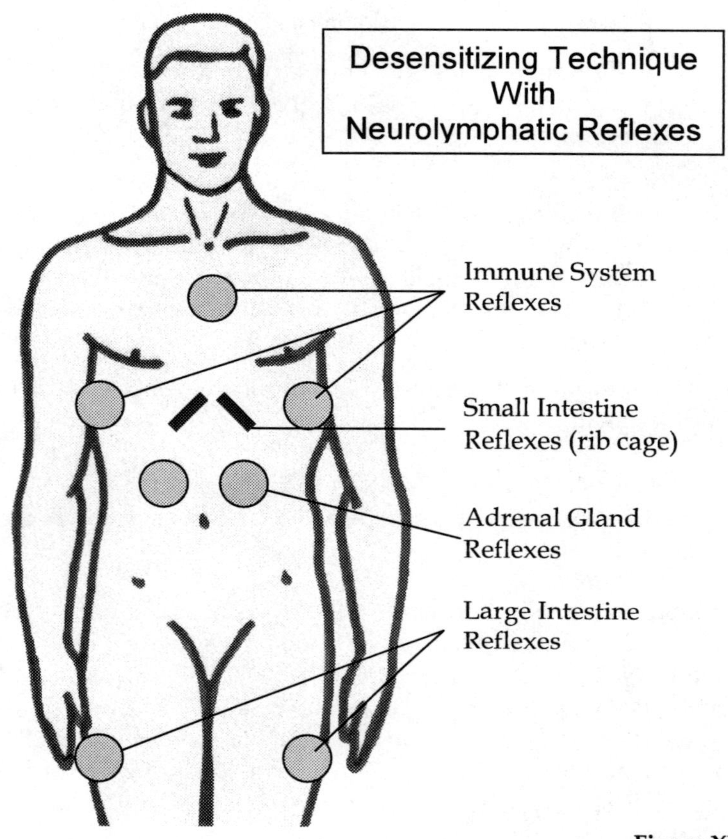

Figure XIV

MISCELLANEOUS

Here are a few other good pieces of information related to the care of your child:

Sore throat - Have your child gargle equal parts salt and baking soda in water. This concoction disrupts the environment in the throat making it difficult for organisms to live.

Common Cold - Keep the immune system strong. Give your child plenty of fresh air and sunshine. Mild exercise like walking can also be very helpful to encourage lymphatic drainage. Keep their diet clean. Do not give them sugar! Sleep is also extremely important because it is the time when our bodies heal. That is one of the reasons why we are so tired when we are sick. Finally, wash your child's hands frequently to prevent the spread of organisms to the rest of the family.

Fungal infections - If your child is chronically sick, has childhood asthma, ADD or ADHD, you should have him checked for a fungal infection. Although chronic conditions have many contributing factors, fungal or other microorganism infections are usually involved.

Fever - When a fever is present it means that your child's body is fighting an organism. I do not believe that you should attempt to alter this reaction with over-the-counter medication unless the fever gets above 104 degrees F. or if your child is prone to febrile seizures. Make sure your child is well hydrated, but do not use juice (unless you make it yourself).

EXERCISE

Technology has allowed for many wondrous things, from life-saving medical advancements to walking on the moon, but it has also made us sedentary. If our occupation does not provide the required amount of exercise then it must be supplemented. Therefore in today's world, the gym may be a necessary place to go to meet our exercise requirements. Numerous studies have shown the beneficial effects of exercise. In fact, proper exercise is one of the keys to the prevention of every known disease. Unfortunately, the topic of exercise can be just as confusing as the topic of diet. Which kind? How much? What about fat burning? These are all common questions. After reading this chapter I hope you will have the answer to these questions and many more.

What Is Exercise?

Exercise can be almost any activity that uses our muscles with a beneficial degree of intensity and for a sustained duration. Do not assume however, that all exercise is equal or that all exercise is beneficial.

What Is The Best Exercise For Our Bodies?

It depends upon our goals. Losing fat, gaining muscle mass, going long distances etc. are all acceptable goals and various forms of exercise can be utilized to achieve them. However, when pursuing the goal of health, only certain forms of exercise, at certain times, are effective. In other words, *a person who is healthy may use all forms of exercise, but not all exercise makes a person healthy.*

FITNESS vs. HEALTH

Before I ever knew anything about exercise, nutrition and the adverse effects of stress, I was able to maintain a high degree of fitness from regular exercise. Basketball and weight lifting were an integral part of my week. If a stranger looked at me, he would think I was in good shape and healthy. Yet, with a sustained increase in stress, I would usually get sick. Other signs were also present, including chronic mucus in my throat, frequent sniffling, sneezing, allergies to cats and dogs and some foods, achy joints, and swelling in my left knee. Although I was able to lift weights for two hours at a time and play basketball half of the day, I was still plagued with the above symptoms. Although I was fit, I was not healthy. I believe that most exercise programs that utilize the "no pain, no gain" approach are unintentionally producing the same problems among the public.

For our purposes, fitness is defined as *adapted to, or suited.* When an athlete allows his body to adapt to the various stressors he has placed upon it, the body will most certainly become fit. Health, however, is defined as *all the systems of the body working together harmoniously and in their most efficient manner.* The fit person is not necessarily healthy, nor is the healthy person necessarily fit. The fit athlete, having trained his body appropriately, is able to perform strenuous and astounding feats, yet this benefit will most likely come at the expense of other tissues, and often of health itself.

It is not uncommon to hear that an athlete has had his career cut short due to nagging injuries, or has even died unexpectantly while training. From my experience and study, I have found that certain deficiencies can be expected when we train for fitness and not for health. These deficiencies often lead to persistent injury, sickness and in extreme cases, death. This is because fitness training places heavy burdens on the body's anaerobic (sugar burning) system, while neglecting the more important aerobic (oxygen and fat burning) system.

THE ANAEROBIC SYSTEM

The anaerobic system is vital to life. It gives us the quick energy we need by using stored glycogen (blood sugar) to perform an activity. Very small amounts of glycogen are available for use by our muscles at any given time. That is why weight training "sets" last only a short period before the muscles, "burn out." Too much anaerobic training can cause chemical imbalances leading to injury and eventually illness. Weight training, sprinting, fast jogging, and most other sports are forms of anaerobic exercise.

Without a doubt, we need our anaerobic systems for burning sugar, brain energy, maintaining fat burning and for an additional source of body energy during times of stress. Also, regular amounts of resistance exercise, like weight training for example, have been shown to strengthen bones and the surrounding soft tissues in women with osteoporosis. There are other benefits as well. Unfortunately an imbalance is present in this society, with too much emphasis placed on anaerobic development.

We are made up of two types of muscle fibers that are simply named "fast" and "slow". Fast fibers are also called anaerobic fibers, while slow fibers are called aerobic fibers. Your genetic makeup often determines how much of each you have. Through training, an athlete can change the function of a particular fiber, making a slow fiber act like a fast fiber and vice versa. Once training has stopped, the cells gradually return to normal. Sprinters and bodybuilders do not have the same number of slow fibers as long distance athletes; instead, they have a great deal more fast fibers. All athletes, which include everyone who exercises regularly, have certain special needs. However, it is interesting to note that athletes participating in fast fiber sports perform better if they train their slow fibers as well according to the method given below.

THE AEROBIC SYSTEM

Aerobic training, (light jogging, easy swimming, easy biking etc.), is extremely beneficial in the promotion of health. In order to engage this system, we must exercise within a certain, low heart rate range. The aerobic system relies on great amounts of oxygen in order to produce energy, and the major fuel used when training aerobically is fat. The same amount of fat contains more than twice as much potential fuel as do carbohydrates. Therefore, when we engage our aerobic systems during exercise, we not only become more efficient, we also burn fat. Not only should fat be our fuel of choice for energy, it is also the one most people want to get rid of in the first place. Too much aerobic training is possible, but rare. For the most part, aerobic activity will strengthen our immune, respiratory, circulatory and musculoskeletal systems. Additionally, we lose fat and increase our energy.

The most appropriate exercise for people is a prolonged, steady use of our slow fibers. Studies examining the effects of aerobic exercise and general health bear this out. Walking and other forms of aerobic exercise have been recommended for all people, because of their health promoting effects.

Benefits of aerobic exercise:

- Decreases stress on sensitive tissues like the adrenal glands
- Reduces the chance of over-training
- Increases blood circulation to all tissues
- Strengthens immune system
- Promotes fat loss
- Detoxifies tissues and eliminates waste

Exercise Goals

It was very difficult for me to give up basketball, even when I knew that the anaerobic stress was damaging my tissues. My love for competition, continued improvement in the sport and overall enjoyment of the game were the reasons I had a hard time quitting. Needless to say, my emotional attachment to the sport allowed for a distortion of my priorities. I had often told patients, concerning their health, "Short term sacrifice means long term benefits," and, "discipline is not a four letter word." Knowing I was not practicing what I preached, and hearing my own words echo in my head, I soon submitted to my conscience. The good news is that once I began to develop my aerobic system, I was able to once again play basketball, and this time without pain.

Many of you who are reading this book may have an emotional attachment to one or several things that are not healthy. You may need to give up some things completely; others may be returned to you in time, once a greater level of health is achieved. You should not look at these changes as anything but positive. Always remember that when we take care of the things God has placed in our trust, including our body, we are blessed.

How to Start

There are two goals with exercise - to care for our bodies, or if you are an athlete, to improve performance. The program below meets both of these goals.

Almost all people have an aerobic system deficiency; those that don't, will not be harmed by doing extra aerobic work. Therefore, we should start by building the aerobic base. This may take up to three months. During this time, NO anaerobic exercise should be performed. For some this may sound difficult, and it is. You will find an appropriate time or season in your schedule. Just remember that exercise is an integral part of health. Without exercise, health is not possible, so the sooner you start, the better.

Dr. Phil Maffetone wrote a book, In Fitness and in Health, which discuses the topic of exercise in depth. I have found this book to be a straight-forward, common-sense approach to exercise and have included many of his ideas in the exercise programs I recommend. I present some of these ideas below.

TARGET HEART RATE

(See: TRACKING SHEETS)

The body switches from fat burning to sugar burning at a specific heart rate. Therefore, the purchase of a heart rate monitor is highly recommended. Once you enter the high heart rate range and engage the anaerobic system you will no longer burn fat even if you return to a lower heart rate. This means that all aerobic benefit could potentially be lost. A heart rate monitor will help you stay below the anaerobic range and will beep when you exceed it. Heart rate monitors are very simple to use and usually include two pieces: a wrist piece that tells the rate of beats per minute (doubles as a watch when not in use) and a strap that goes around the chest which picks up the electrical signal given off by the heart. They may be purchased at most sports stores for less than $100.00.

To find your target heart rate range:

1. **Take 180 and subtract your age.**
2. **Then add or subtract from this number based upon the following:**
   - Recovering from a major illness, surgery or taking daily medication.....**subtract 10**
   - Have not exercised before, or have exercised but have been injured or are regressing, or experience frequent colds, flu, or under high stress.....**subtract 5**
   - Exercising for up to two years without any real problems, and have not had colds or flu more than once or twice per year.....**subtract 0**
   - Exercising for more than two years without any real problems and have been making progress in your program or competition.....**add 5**

For example, a fifty year old man who rarely exercises and gets the flu and/or a cold or two most years would have a maximum aerobic heart rate of 125bpm (180 - 50 -5). Then, his maximum aerobic range would be from ten beats below his maximum, up to his maximum (115bpm-125bpm). The heart rate monitor can be set for this range. When exercising above or below this range, a beep will sound.

Without A Heart Rate Monitor

You will still derive great benefit from training your aerobic system, even if it is below the ideal range, and you will lose some benefit when the range is exceeded. So, exercise at a very low pace. A light sweat, easy breathing and a feeling of not having done much when through are all good signs that indicate you have trained below your maximum rate.

What to Expect

Most people will be shocked at how quickly their heart rate exceeds their maximum range. I frequently need to reinforce this style of exercise to patients who simply can't believe that training so slowly can do any good. Patients who are presently joggers and who exercised two or three times per week with no apparent difficulty, are surprised to find that their normal exercise routine produced a heart rate 10, 20, 30 or more beats above maximum. These were the same patients who showed many signs of adrenal fatigue and nagging injuries. In only a short period of time, after training in their aerobic range, they were able to resume their previous running course and speed, this time with a much lower heart rate and few, if any, nagging injuries. This indicated that they had indeed developed their aerobic base and were beginning to receive its many benefits.

Another sign that you are training aerobically is the presence of sore muscles. Since most people have trained their fast fibers while neglecting their slow fibers, they have unknowingly become sugar burners instead of fat burners. While training at a lower heart rate, the slow (fat burning) fibers will be the primary tissues worked, leading to soreness. This soreness, after an easy aerobic workout, is good. It will pass in a few days and is a sign that you are on the right track.

Selecting a Program

An aerobic program should be performed at least three times per week for thirty minutes each time. As the training progresses, frequency (up to five, sometimes six times per week) and time (up to sixty minutes or more) can be increased.

Walking is the best way to start and will be the only choice for most people. If you are currently doing some form of exercise, then your body may be able to lightly jog or swim. Whatever the exercise, it should involve the large muscles of the legs, be continuous for the determined amount of time and always stay in or below the target heart rate range.

THE EMOTIONAL COMPONENT

Wanting to exercise can be just as important as doing it. The emotional component in any activity should always be addressed. Therefore, pick a route that is enjoyable, a time of day that is convenient, clothing that is comfortable, and an attitude that is appreciative and determined. Tying productive emotions into any new routine or discipline helps to get through the tougher stages and encourages progress.

WARM UP, COOL DOWN AND STRETCHING

Warming up and stretching are essential, but they are not the same thing and should not be done at the same time. Warming up is as simple as a slow easy walk for ten minutes. It is necessary in order to prepare the body for exercise. Warming up should always be done first. Once exercise begins, the metabolic by-products (toxins) of muscle activity need somewhere to go. Warming up ensures that a sufficient amount of blood is circulating prior to exercise, so that these by-products can be carried away to the liver for detoxification and elimination. Warming up also increases the amount of free-floating fatty acids available for fuel - our desired energy source. Also, up to 80% of the blood in the organs will be transferred to the muscles during stressful activity. Warming up allows for this to happen slowly and gradually, decreasing the overall amount of tissue stress. Ten to fifteen minutes is all that is required for a proper warm up period.

After a brief warm up period, stretching may be performed. The added circulation from the warm up period allows for greater elasticity and flexibility of the tissues during a stretch, both of which decrease the chance for injury. Do not stretch through the point of pain and do not bounce when you stretch. Stretching beyond the normal range of motion may temporarily increase flexibility, but it also leads to micro injury. The best form of stretching is a static-active stretch. This means that you perform a light stretch, moving slowly to a point of resistance, and contract the opposite muscle for 10-20 seconds. For example, if you want to stretch the muscles on the back of the right leg, mildly contract the muscles on the front of the right leg for about 20 seconds.

The cool down is just as important as the warm up. Cooling down allows a gentle return of the blood to the various organs. If we stop suddenly after exercise, the blood rushes too quickly into the organs, bringing with it the many chemical waste products that were produced. Since most of our blood is stored in the organs when we are not active, many of the chemical waste products will be trapped there as well. This leads to chemical stress and potential toxic buildup. If severe enough, all the aerobic benefits from the exercise can be lost. Also, the cool down is the first stage of the post-exercise recovery. Recovery from exercise is just as important as the exercise itself. Simply go gradually slower than the exercise pace until your heart rate is about 10 - 20 beats above your resting heart rate. This should only take about ten minutes and is all that is needed.

You will begin to get to know more about your body and its specific needs before, during and after exercise. Always try to, "tune in," to what is going on in your tissues as you exercise. The body gives us many warning signs; we need only to pay attention and heed its call.

MAXIMUM AEROBIC FUNCTION TEST (MAF)
(see: TRACKING SHEETS)
After beginning an exercise program, it is important to monitor progress to ensure that you are developing as intended. You will notice many subjective changes: feeling better, not as tired, more energy, not as sick, sleeping better etc. Also, you should perform a maximum aerobic function test (MAF) to check for objective changes as well.

Pick a distance that can be measured. When you begin the program, while walking in your target heart rate range, complete your chosen course and record your time. Over the next few weeks repeat the test. If you are able to walk the same distance in less time while maintaining your target heart rate range then you are improving your aerobic system. The opposite can be done as well. Pick an amount of time you are going to perform an exercise, and measure how far you go. If you are making progress, you should be able to go further in the same amount of time on the next test. These tests are important emotionally because they demonstrate that progress is being made, which encourages further exercise. Perform an MAF test every 3 or 4 weeks.

If you are not improving, evaluate your health. Have you been sick, stressed, getting enough rest, eating bad foods etc.? Address these issues and keep going. Most will find that they improve rather quickly and that they have to progress from walking to a slow jog in order to maintain their minimum heart rate range.

Summary

- Train aerobically for three months without anaerobic exercise.
- Do not exceed your maximum heart rate at any time during your workout.
- When training without a heart rate monitor, only exercise at a pace where little exertion is noticed.
- Warm up.
- Stretch.
- Cool down.
- Do monthly MAF tests to ensure progress.

When to Add Other Exercises

After the initial three months is over, you may begin adding back your favorite exercises as long as they are the minority activity of your week. Aerobic exercise will always be the best for our bodies because that is how we were designed. You should find however, that after an initial adjustment period, you are now able to perform your old exercises at an even greater level of ease and comfort. In a two-week period, I may play basketball once or twice, lift weights two to four times and do aerobic training in between. I do these activities because I find them enjoyable, and this regimen seems to work well for me.

SELF TREATMENT

Occasionally, I get a request from someone elsewhere in the country or overseas asking if I could design a program to help them overcome their illness. If a qualified practitioner in their area cannot be found or if they insist on a program specifically from me, I agree to help. Below, I describe what I call a neuro-immune treatment (NIT). It is an at-home program designed to help reduce the sensitivity of the immune system to various organisms, foods or chemicals. Along with this program I make sure to include specific supplements, and information on diet and exercise. I know which supplements and lifestyle recommendations to make based upon their answers to an extensive health questionnaire.

This protocol is designed primarily to help with chronic or longstanding conditions. All longstanding conditions have a nutritional component. This means that the proper nutrients will aid in recovery. In addition, most chronic conditions have a microbial component. In other words, they are in one way or another related to the presence or absence of certain microorganisms (bacteria, viruses, yeast etc.). If a microorganism is present a sample will always be found in stool. In our office, when the stool is tested with applied kinesiology (AK), a patient's strong test muscle will weaken if there is a disease-promoting organism (see: SECTION I: Applied Kinesiology). The patient will also weaken to foods that they are allergic to, or any other adverse stimuli.

NIT, as stated above, is a desensitization protocol. The nervous and immune systems often become sensitive to a substance that has either been eaten too often for too long, or in the case of microorganisms, has been contracted (i.e. parasites) or grown out of proportion (i.e. Candidiasis). I discuss how desensitization works in SECTION II: Allergies.

Long-standing conditions include:

- Pain
    - Arthritis
    - Headaches/Migraines
    - Nerve Pain
- Infections
    - Viral (Epstein-Barr)
    - Fungal (Candidiasis)
    - Parasitic
    - Bacterial
- Allergies
    - Airborne Allergies
    - Chemical Sensitivities
    - Food Allergies
- Digestive Problems
    - Constipation
    - Crohn's Disease
    - G.E.R.D.
    - Irritable Bowel Disease
    - Ulcerative Colitis
    - Weight Gain
- Chronic Conditions
    - Chronic Fatigue
    - Fibromyalgia
    - Multiple Sclerosis
    - Organ Deficiencies
- Reproductive Conditions
    - Enlarged Prostate
    - Fibroids
    - Ovarian Cysts

NIT PROTOCOL

Perform this protocol twice a day for three weeks. You can go longer or perform it more often if you would like. Remember, to achieve the best results with NIT, lifestyle changes in the form of a proper diet and exercise are essential.

What you will need:

- A comfortable place to lie down
- A small towel
- Stool Sample
- Neurolymphatic Chart
- Beginning & Ending Points Chart

Before beginning, read through these instructions in order to familiarize yourself with the NIT protocol.

STEP I - COLLECT A BODY SAMPLE

Collection: A very small amount of stool is all that is needed. Simply take an old supplement bottle or other clean container. After a bowel movement, place the toilet paper that you used to wipe with into the jar. This toilet paper will contain enough of a sample for testing. Seal the container tightly. If possible, try to collect the sample the day you perform the NIT protocol. If you do not have daily bowel movements, simply store the sample somewhere safe (away from children or spouses) and reuse it the following day.

STEP II – SAMPLE PLACEMENT

Lie comfortably on your back. Place the sample on your abdomen and cover with a small towel (this makes sure that the supplement does not roll off). You want to make sure that your arms can freely move about without losing the sample.

STEP III – THE EMOTIONAL COMPONENT

Longstanding illnesses always carry with them an emotional component. We address this by having you think of how you have felt at your worst with this problem. Try to be specific. If there was pain, think of the kind of pain (sharp, burning, aching etc.). If there is digestive distress, try to think of the details of those symptoms (bloated feeling, stomach churning etc.) Try to think of these negative thoughts for each of the treatment steps until it is time to repeat. When you repeat the treatment sequence, you will now think of a positive thought (see: Step VI). With the sample in place and the proper thought in your mind, you are now ready to begin NIT.

STEP IV – TREATING THE NEUROLYMPHATIC REFLEXES

Look at the chart of the Neurolymphatic Reflexes. Rub each set of reflexes for about 20 or 30 seconds. It is not necessary to be overly vigorous or precise. Rubbing the general area will do. You may rub each matching pair at the same time using one hand for each side. There is an additional small intestine reflex on each wrist. This reflex needs to be tapped in the same manner as the tapping performed in Step V.

STEP V – TREATING THE BEGINNING & ENDING POINTS

Look at the chart of the Beginning & Ending points. Like the previous reflexes, there are matching pairs that generally relate to a specific organ. Tap each of these points with one or two fingers (two fingers, such as the index and middle finger, may ensure that you hit the right spot). The tapping should last 15 or 20 seconds. It does not need to be vigorous.

STEP VI – REPEAT STEPS IV & V

Now that you have made it through, repeat the same steps, this time remembering to think of a positive thought. For instance, think of a time that you were very strong and active. Or, tell yourself with enthusiasm that you will soon be well. Here are some examples:

- "I am overcoming my illness and will be completely restored to health."
- "This protocol is working to make me better."

If you find that you are having trouble believing that you will get well, you should say something like:

- "I choose only to believe that I will soon be well."
- "I dismiss all thoughts that would prevent me from becoming healthy."

That's it! It may seem strange or unimpressive but it works. Remember to perform this protocol twice a day and don't forget about the important lifestyle changes that support NIT.

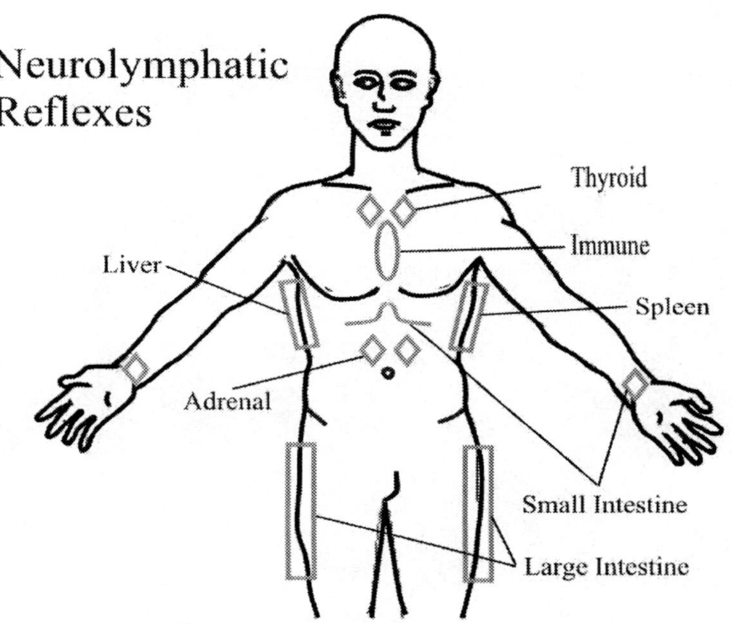

Figure XV

- **Thyroid** – located just below the collar bone where it attaches to the breast bone
- **Immune** – located along the entire breast bone
- **Small Intestine** – located at the lower margin of the rib cage and at the center of the wrist
- **Liver** – located along the right side of the torso and under the right breast
- **Spleen** – located along the left side of the torso and under the left breast
- **Adrenal** – located 2 cm up and 2 cm over from the belly button
- **Large Intestine** – located along the outside of the legs from just below the hips to the side of the knee.

BEGINNING AND ENDING POINTS

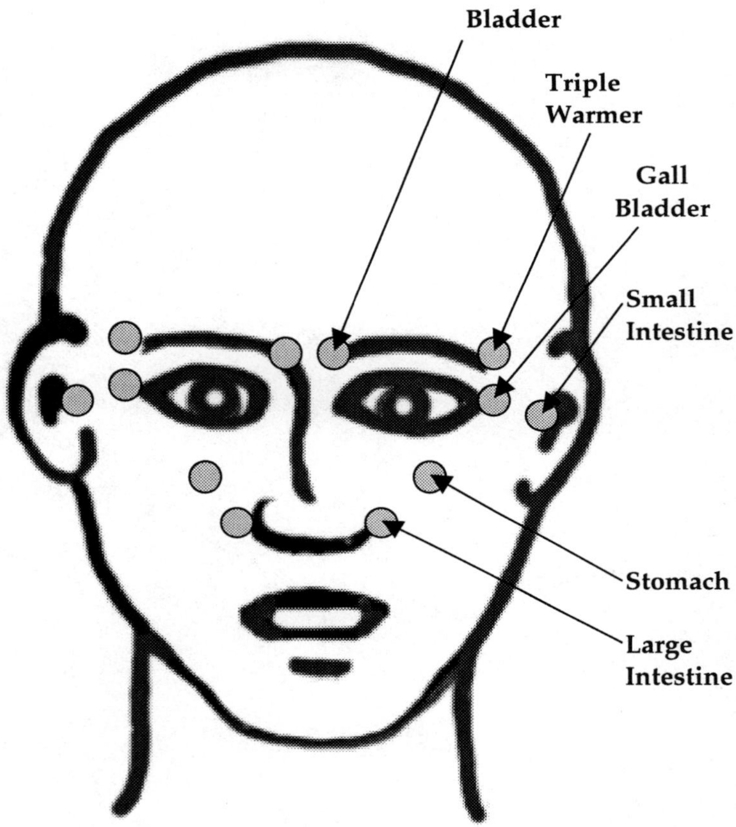

Figure XVI

- **Bladder** – located where the nose and eyebrows begin
- **Triple Warmer** – located at the under edge of the eyebrows
- **Gall Bladder** – located at the outer edge of the eyes
- **Small Intestine** – located in front of the ear hole
- **Stomach** – located 2cm below the eye
- **Large Intestine** – located at the widest aspects of the nose

RESOURCES

SECTION IV

YEAST DIET

Dietary Recommendations:
The dietary recommendations given below are designed to work in conjunction with a nutritional protocol and with in-office treatments. In some cases it may be necessary to strictly adhere to the diet below. Some people are so sensitive to intestinal yeast infections that any wavering from the recommended diet will result in re-infection.

Eat:

- Meats: beef, duck, eggs, quail, chicken, fish, oyster, rabbit, clam, tuna, turkey, crab, shrimp, goose, pheasant, lobster, Cornish hen, lamb, pork, and veal.
- Vegetables (excluding corn and potatoes) asparagus, broccoli, cauliflower, eggplant, parsley, zucchini squash, avocado, brussel sprouts, celery, green pepper, peas, tomatoes, green beans, yellow beans, cabbage, okra, beets, carrots, cucumber, onion, radishes, greens: beet, collard, kale, lettuce, mustard, spinach & turnip.
- Nuts: almonds, Brazil nuts, cashews, filberts, pecans, and walnuts.
- Seed: sesame seeds, sunflower seeds, and pumpkin seeds.
- Oils: butter, almond, avocado, canola, corn, flax, olive, sesame, sunflower.
- Brown rice
- Avocado
- Millet

- Quinoa pasta
- Live yogurt (plain)
- Water lemon and grapefruit juice (freshly squeezed only)
- Kefir (a fermented beverage made from whole milk)
- Dairy: whole milk, unaged cheese, cream. Dairy products should be eaten hot. This is important. Unsalted butter and plain yogurt are less of a problem than the other dairy products.
- Miscellaneous: I do not like to recommend these less-than-vital foods. Some may even be harmful. However, for the short term, for taste, and in order to rid the patient of Candida as quickly as possible, I make these exceptions. Nutrasweet®, Equal®, Jell-O®, rice cakes, sesame rice crackers, Triscuits®, Shredded Wheat®, raw unpasteurized apple cider vinegar, Stevia (available at health food stores). This is a controversial section.

Do Not Eat: These foods cause Candida to grow.

- **Sugars** (see the bottom of the Maintenance & Prevention Diet): honey, molasses, maple syrup, corn syrup, dextrose, sorbitol.
- Aged cheeses
- Alcohol
- Chocolate
- Citrus fruits (except grapefruit and lemon)
- Dried fruits
- Fermented foods
- Wheat
- Oats
- Rye
- Barley
- Ham

- Nut butters
- Processed & smoked meats
- Raw mushrooms
- Soy sauce
- Sprouts
- All yeast products
- All "sweet" drinks.
- Leftovers (usually contain molds)
- Vinegar-containing foods (catsup, mustard, mayonnaise, salad dressings, pickles)

Snack: If you substitute whole-wheat flour for white, carob chips for chocolate chips, butter for margarine (you should do that anyway) and Nutrasweet® for sugar you can make delicious cookies. Eat these cookies hot and in small amounts, but don't forget to do everything else.

Avoid:

- Antibiotics and steroid drugs (e.g.. birth control pills).
- Chemicals: household products and cleaners, chlorinated water, mothballs, moldy places.
- Other: Use a new toothbrush every three weeks to prevent re-infection. Also, fungus may be spread through the saliva, so sexual contact with another fungal carrier may slow the recovery.

Give yourself at least two months on this program. Remember, you have probably had Candida for a very long time and you will be susceptible to it again in the future if you let your guard down. Don't be surprised if in a few months you again feel badly after eating cinnamon rolls and ice cream or any other sugar snack. Recognize your weaknesses and be smart.

RECIPES

All of the following recipes have low amounts of carbohydrates. This means that they are acceptable for those on a high protein diet or a sugar avoidance diet. For those on an anti-yeast diet, some ingredients are not permitted. Simply check the recipe and substitute a recommended food in place of the non-recommended food (see: Yeast Diet).

Almost any recipe can be modified to suit your particular restriction. Soups, salads and stews are easily modified recipes. You can use different meats, vegetables and toppings while staying within your guidelines. Herbs and spices add terrific taste to an otherwise dull meal. Use these liberally.

Most of these recipes were found on various websites, which are listed under the recipe name. Be sure to check our resources as well. Here are the recipes contained within this chapter:

EGGS
Cheese Artichoke Oven Omelet
Spinach "Pancake"
Spinach-Filled Stuffed Eggs
Ham Stuffed Eggs
Asparagus Frittata

PORK & TURKEY
Cured Pork Shoulder
Roasted Turkey with herbs

CHICKEN
Whole Roasted Chicken
Chicken Ham Bake
Chicken a la Tom
Chicken with Pesto
Fried Chicken

SOUPS
Ham and Bean Soup
Egg Drop Soup
Dilled Vegetable Soup
Non-Dairy Creamy Soup
Lentil Soup

SALADS
Hot Spinach Salad
Tangy Warm Chicken Salad
Chicken Salad
Tabouli Salad
Tahini Chicken Salad

BEEF
Beef and Broccoli Stir Fry
Hearty Beef Stew

OTHERS
Basic Salad Dressing
Caesar Salad Dressing
Mayonnaise

EGGS

CHEESE ARTICHOKE OVEN OMELET

Melissa Martin

- 1 cup of salsa
- 1 can of artichoke hearts (or other veggies or meats)
- Your favorite cheeses
- 5-7 eggs
- ¼ cup sour cream

Grease a 9" pie plate. Spread salsa in the bottom, enough to cover. On top of the salsa spread a can of artichoke hearts, broken into pieces. Over that spread a variety of shredded cheeses (I like parmesan, extra sharp white cheddar, I even tried havarti with dill once and it was wonderful), as little or as much as you like. In a separate bowl beat together 5-7 eggs and the sour cream. Pour mixture over the cheese, bake at 350 degrees until set and lightly browned on top.

SPINACH "PANCAKE"

www.lowcarb.com

- 4 T unsalted butter
- 4 green onions, thinly sliced
- 1/4 cup chopped fresh parsley
- 1/2 lb. spinach, washed and stemmed
- 3 eggs
- Sea salt and freshly ground black pepper
- Sour cream for serving, if desired

Melt 3 Tbsp. of the butter in a large frying pan over medium heat. Add the green onions and parsley and cook until the onion wilts. Add the spinach and cook, stirring until it wilts. Turn the heat to low and cook, stirring occasionally for 20 minutes. The spinach will become quite soft and smooth.

Beat the eggs and stir in the spinach mixture. Season to taste. Melt the remaining butter in a 10-inch, preferably nonstick frying pan over medium high heat. Spread out the spinach mixture in the pan. Cover, turn the heat to medium low and cook for 10 minutes or until set. Serve with sour cream if you like.

SPINACH-FILLED STUFFED EGGS

www.lowcarbluxury.com

- 12 hard-cooked eggs
- 1 (10-ounce) package frozen chopped spinach or 1 bunch fresh spinach, cooked and chopped
- 1/4 cup organic mayonnaise
- 2 T olive oil
- 2 T freshly grated parmesan cheese
- Salt and freshly ground pepper to taste

Cook the spinach. Drain and squeeze dry, getting out as much water as possible so spinach doesn't dilute the filling.

Peel eggs and cut in half. Mash yolks with spinach, mayonnaise, oil, cheese, salt and pepper. Carefully fill each egg white half with the yolk mixture. Cover with plastic wrap and refrigerate until well chilled.

HAM STUFFED EGGS

www.lowcarbluxury.com

- 6 hard-cooked eggs
- 3 to 4 T mayonnaise (see below)
- 2 teaspoons Dijon mustard
- 2 to 3 T finely minced ham
- Salt and freshly ground pepper to taste

Peel eggs and cut each egg in half. Remove the yolks and mash with mayonnaise and mustard. Stir in ham until well combined. Season to taste with salt and pepper. Fill each egg white half with mixture. Cover with plastic wrap and refrigerate until well chilled.

ASPARAGUS FRITTATA

www.lowcarbluxury.com

- 12 asparagus spears *
- 8 large eggs
- 1/4 cup whipping cream, divided
- 1 t grated lemon peel
- salt to taste
- cayenne to taste
- 1/2 cup grated parmesan cheese
- shredded cheddar cheese (optional)

In a wide frying pan, bring about 1 inch water to a boil over high heat. Meanwhile, snap off and discard tough ends of asparagus; then cut spears into 1-inch pieces. Add asparagus to boiling water and cook, uncovered, until just tender when pierced (3 to 5 minutes), or to your tenderness preference. Drain well.

Divide asparagus among 4 well-buttered 4 to 5 inch-wide ovenproof dishes. Carefully break 2 eggs over asparagus in each dish. Spoon 1 tablespoon of the cream over eggs in each dish. Then sprinkle eggs evenly with lemon peel, and with salt and cayenne to taste.

Set dishes on a baking sheet and bake in a 450° oven until eggs are done to your liking (5 to 7 minutes for firm whites and soft yolks). Sprinkle evenly with cheese and bake for 1 more minute. Serve at once. (If you are using the cheddar cheese sprinkles as well, add them after the parmesan extra baking minute and give it 1-2 more minutes to melt and bubble.)

* *Stalking Fresh Asparagus* - You may think peeled asparagus is a tedious affectation. But first, consider the benefits. Without that fibrous exterior, you can enjoy each spear to its tender base. Here's how to do it with the least fuss. First snap off and discard the tough ends of the asparagus. Then, holding the spear near the tip, peel away scales and the thin outer skin. An ordinary vegetable peeler works best, and one glide per cut will do; there's no need to whittle away at the stalk. Peeling goes faster than you think, especially if you look for the fattest asparagus when you shop.

PORK & TURKEY

CURED PORK SHOULDER

www.lowcarb.com

The slow-roasting and dry marinade makes the pork very tender and succulent. It's just fantastic cold.

- 1 4-5 lb. boneless, skinless pork shoulder, not rolled or tied
- 2 T coriander seeds
- 1 T whole black peppercorns
- 12 whole cloves
- 1 T sea salt
- 2 bay leaves, crumbled
- 2 T fresh rosemary leaves, coarsely chopped
- 6 cloves garlic, thinly sliced

With a sharp knife, score the pork fat in a cross-hatch pattern.

Combine the coriander seeds, peppercorns and cloves in a coffee grinder or mortar and pestle. Grind coarsely and combine with the salt, bay leaves, rosemary and garlic. Spread half the mixture in the bottom of a glass or non-corrodible pan and place the pork on top. Cover with the remaining mixture. Cover and refrigerate overnight.

Preheat the oven to 250°F. Wash the pork and pat dry. Place fat side up in a baking pan and bake for 6 hours - that's right, 6 hours. Let rest for 15 minutes before slicing.

ROASTED TURKEY WITH HERBS

www.lowcarb.com

- 1 15 lb. (7 kg) turkey
- ½ lb. pancetta (Italian ham/bacon)
- ½ cup fresh rosemary leaves
- 4 whole heads garlic
- 6 cloves garlic, minced
- ½ t salt

- 1 t coarsely ground black pepper
- olive oil
- 2 cups dry red wine
- ½ cup finely chopped shallots

Preheat the oven to 350 F. Rinse the turkey and pat dry. Finely chop half the pancetta and cut the other half into large chunks. Stuff the large chunks of pancetta, half the rosemary leaves and the whole heads of garlic into the cavity of the turkey. Transfer the finely chopped pancetta to a food processor with the remaining rosemary, minced garlic, salt and pepper. Pulse until everything is finely chopped.

Loosen the skin of the turkey over the breast and around the legs. Slide the pancetta mixture over the breast and legs, under the skin, patting it out evenly. Transfer to a roasting pan and rub the turkey with olive oil. Tie the legs loosely.

Roast for 3-3½ hours basting the turkey with ½ cup (120 ml) of the red wine every 30 minutes. After the second basting, scatter the shallots in the bottom of the roasting pan.

Remove the turkey from the roasting pan. Degrease the juices with a fat separator or skim with a spoon. Strain through a sieve into a pot; keep warm over low heat and adjust the seasoning. Remove the whole garlic from the cavity and separate the cloves. Carve the turkey into slices and garnish with the cloves of garlic, which are meant to be eaten. Serve with the pan juices on the side.

SALADS

TANGY WARM CHICKEN SALAD

www.lowcarbluxury.com

- 1/4 cup (1/2 stick) butter, divided
- 2 whole chicken breasts (skinned, boned and cut into thin strips)
- 1/3 cup chopped red pepper
- 1 cup cooked asparagus pieces
- 2 T minced shallots
- 1 teaspoon dried tarragon (or 1 tablespoon fresh tarragon, minced.)
- 1 cup whipping cream
- 1 T Dijon-style prepared mustard
- 1/4 cup toasted almonds

Over low heat, melt 2 tablespoons butter in large skillet. Sauté chicken pieces until cooked throughout. Meanwhile, melt remaining 2 tablespoons butter in medium-sized skillet. Cook red pepper, asparagus, shallots and tarragon over medium heat until vegetables are tender, about 5 minutes. Set aside. Add whipping cream to chicken. Heat to boiling, stirring frequently. Reduce heat to low, stirring constantly until cream is reduced and thickened, about 5 minutes. Stir in vegetable mixture and mustard, cooking until thoroughly heated. Sprinkle with almonds and serve immediately.

HOT SPINACH SALAD

www.lowcarbluxury.com

- 1 pound fresh young spinach,
- (coarse stems discarded and leaves washed well and spun dry)
- 1/4 cup sliced green onions
- 5 slices bacon
- 1/4 cup balsamic vinegar

- 2 hard boiled eggs (sliced)
- Sweetener to taste
- salt and pepper to taste

Shred spinach into bowl. Add onions. Chop bacon; fry until crisp; add vinegar, seasoning & sweetener. Heat to boiling; pour quickly over spinach mixture. Toss until wilted. Garnish with egg slices.

CHICKEN SALAD

Kristin
(world's greatest office manager)

- Shredded cooked chicken breast
- Crushed Garlic
- Fresh lemon juice
- Tahini
- Cilantro
- Favorite Greens

In mini chopper blend everything except the chicken. Mix ingredients with shredded chicken and put on a bed of your favorite greens.

TABOULI SALAD

- 3 cups sprouts
- 1 cup parsley, minced
- ½ cup onion, minced
- 2 ripe tomatoes, chopped
- 2 t dried mint or basil (or ¼ cup fresh herbs)
- 2 lemons, juiced
- ¼ cup olive oil
- garlic powder
- pepper to taste

Mix all ingredients together and season to taste with garlic powder and pepper. Let sit for ½ hour or more to blend flavors. Serve on lettuce leaves.

TAHINI CHICKEN SALAD

- 2 whole boneless skinless chicken breasts
- 8 oz. chicken stock
- ½ - 1 cup water
- 1 cup of Tahini (sesame seed) paste
- 2/3 cup fresh lemon juice
- 2 cloves of garlic
- 1 cup chopped cilantro
- salt & pepper
- 1 whole tomato
- 1/3 cup lightly toasted pine nuts

Poach the chicken in chicken stock and water until done. Cool slightly and shred. Set aside in a large bowl. In a blender, mince the garlic, and then add Tahini paste and lemon juice. Blend while adding water until it reaches a desired consistency. Add cilantro. Mix all ingredients with chicken. Season with fresh salt and black pepper to taste. Serve in half a tomato on a bed of greens with pine nuts on top.

CHICKEN

TOM'S WHOLE ROASTED CHICKEN

www.camcdonald.com

Take a whole chicken, split it down the back, taking out most of the upper backbone. Salt & pepper it.

In a fairly shallow pan, place aromatic vegetables, such as celery, carrots, onions, etc. (You don't necessarily have to eat them). Place the chicken, breasts up on top of the veggies. Stuff fresh herbs under the skin, such as basil, oregano, rosemary, tarragon, whatever. Place in a hot oven (400) for about 20 min/pound.

CHICKEN HAM BAKE

www.lowcarb.com

- 4 chicken breasts
- 4 long slices of thin ham
- 4 slices of mozzarella cheese (or Swiss)
- 1 cup of chicken stock (usually two T of stock to 1 cup of water)
- 2 t garlic powder

Place chicken in a baking dish, pour chicken stock over the top, then garlic powder. Cook in preheated 350 degree oven for about an hour. Take chicken out of oven and drain all the stock out of the pan and wrap ham around breast and lay cheese on top. Put back in the oven for another 5 min. Let cool for 5 minutes and enjoy.

CHICKEN A LA TOM

www.lowcarbcafe.com

- 3 boneless, skinless chicken breasts (pounded)
- 3 cloves fresh garlic, minced
- 3 t butter

- 1/4 cup olive oil
- 8 oz. crabmeat (pre-cooked)
- shredded parmesan cheese (optional)
- 1/4 cup white wine (optional)
- fresh spinach
- salt/pepper to taste

Pound the chicken breasts, then salt and pepper if desired. Grill chicken breasts: cut into pieces and set aside. Sautee the garlic in a medium skillet with the butter, olive oil, and wine. Place chicken and crabmeat into skillet. Cook on low/med heat, for 5 min, stirring constantly. To serve, place chicken on a bed of spinach leaves with Parmesan cheese grated over the top.

CHICKEN WITH PESTO

www.lowcarbcafe.com

- 3 cups basil leaves + extra
- 1 cup olive oil + extra
- 1/2 cup pine nuts
- 3/4 cup grated parmesan cheese
- 4 cloves garlic
- 6 chicken breasts (boneless, skinless)
- 1/2 lemon
- salt & pepper to taste

Pesto: Place garlic, 3 cups basil leaves, pine nuts, and enough olive oil to blend well into blender (usually 3/4-1 cup for this many leaves).

Blend on chop or puree to a smooth consistency. Move leaves with spoon if needed. Add parmesan cheese and blend to mix.

Freeze 1/2 the pesto for another time - it freezes well.

Chicken: Slice the breasts into 1 inch strips for quick cooking. Sauté in 2T olive oil. Add lemon juice, salt and pepper. You can add a little wine or broth if liquid is needed.

When chicken is cooked, add another handful of basil leaves. When basil is wilted, remove from heat and add the pesto (approx 3/4 cup) to coat the chicken to your liking.

FRIED CHICKEN
www.lowcarbcafe.com

This is not the healthiest dinner, but after two weeks on the anti-yeast diet you don't mind too much.

- 25 Pieces Pork Rinds
- 1 egg, beaten
- 4 Boneless/Skinless Chicken Breasts

Preheat oven to 400 degrees. Put pork rinds into a sealed plastic bag. Crush the rinds into small crumbs. Dip chicken into egg then drop into plastic bag. Shake to coat. Place on baking sheet and bake for 20-25 minutes or until chicken is done all the way through.

SOUPS

HAM AND BEAN SOUP

www.lowcarbluxury.com

- 8 oz cubed ham
- 1/4 cup finely diced celery
- 1 cup water
- 1 cup low-sodium chicken broth
- 1 can black soy beans
- 1/4 cup tiny diced carrot
- 2 teaspoons minced onion
- 1/4 t minced garlic (optional)
- 1/8 t Cayenne Pepper
- 1/4 t Cumin
- 1/4 t Salt

In a medium sauce pan brown the ham. Add 1 cup of water and scrape glaze off bottom of pan. Add low-sodium chicken broth.

Drain the water from the can of beans. Add beans to the sauce pan.

Add all other ingredients. Stir. Bring to a boil; turn down heat and simmer for at least 1 hour to bring out the flavors -- the longer, the better (3+ hours being best.)

EGG DROP SOUP

www.lowcarbluxury.com

- 2 ½ quarts chicken broth
- 2 T soy sauce
- ¼ Cup chopped green onion
- 4 eggs - slightly beaten
- 1 T Potato Starch (optional)

Combine first 3 ingredients in a large saucepan, bring to a boil. If using potato starch (to thicken a bit), mix it with 2 Tbsp cool water and add slowly to hot broth at this point. Stir to thicken. Slowly pour eggs into the boiling broth. Cook for 1 minute. Serve immediately.

DILLED VEGETABLE SOUP

- 4 cups vegetable stock
- 1 t dill weed
- 1 dash pepper
- 1 ½ cups potatoes; diced
- ½ cup onion, diced
- 3 carrots, sliced – ¼ inch thick
- 2 cups zucchini, sliced
- 2 tomatoes, chopped
- salt to taste

Combine the stock with the dill weed, pepper, potatoes, onion, and carrots in a 2-quart saucepan. Bring the mixture to a full boil, partially cover, reduce the heat and simmer for 20 minutes. Add the zucchini and tomatoes and cook another 10 minutes or until all of the vegetables are tender. Salt to taste and serve hot.

NON- DAIRY CREAMY SOUP

Kristin S.

- 4 Red Peppers (or small bag of baby carrots)
- ½ T olive oil
- 2 crushed garlic cloves
- 2 cans of low sodium chicken stock
- Herbs and spices

Roast & peel the red peppers or steam baby carrots. Mix in a blender until they are a smooth paste. In a soup pan, put in olive oil and crushed garlic cloves – sauté until just before brown. Add the low sodium chicken stock. Add herbs or spices to taste and pureed vegetables. With stick blender, mix thoroughly. Heat to desired temp and serve.

LENTIL SOUP

- 1 lb. sliced smoked sausage (large link)
- 1 lb. lentils
- ½ cup chopped onion
- ½ cup sliced celery
- 1/2 cup sliced carrots
- 1/8 t garlic salt
- 2 1/2 t salt
- 1 1/2 t oregano
- 6 oz can tomato paste
- 8 cups water
- 20 oz can tomatoes

In a large stock pot, combine all of the ingredients except the tomatoes. Cook for 1 hour and 30 minutes. Add the tomatoes and simmer for 30 minutes.

BEEF

BEEF AND BROCCOLI STIR FRY

Dr. Monk

This recipe is easily modified to fit other meats like chicken or shrimp. Try adding different vegetables as well.

- 1 T olive oil
- 2 cups broccoli -- blanched
- 1/2 cup thinly sliced carrot
- 1/2 cup onion -- wedges
- 6 ounces sirloin steak -- boneless, strips
- 1 ½ T chicken broth -- or broth
- 1 t soy sauce, low sodium
- 1/8 t sea salt -- optional
- ½ -1 T arrow root (for thickness)

In a 10" skillet or wok heat the oil; add the prepared vegetables. Cook, stirring quickly & frequently until veggies are crisp tender & onions are browned. Stir in the beef strips and cook until done.

In a small bowl, combine the remaining ingredients, beginning with 1 teaspoon of arrow root. Add this to the beef mixture and while stirring constantly for 2 -3 minutes. If more thickness is desired, an additional teaspoon of arrow root may be used.

If you are not on an anti-yeast diet, then you can also add in 1-2 tablespoons of honey for sweetness.

HEARTY BEEF STEW

Kristin (world's greatest office manager)

- 2 lbs. stew beef
- 2 cloves crushed garlic
- 1 T olive oil
- 1 medium onion

- 1 large can crushed tomatoes
- 1 small can of tomato paste
- 1 can vegetable or beef broth
- Baby carrots (1 package)
- New potatoes (1/2 - 1 pound)
- 1 regular package of button mushrooms (quartered)
- 1 portabella mushroom (in chunks)
- Sea salt and pepper
- Basil
- Balsamic vinegar
- Oregano
- 1 T corn starch

Brown the meat in olive oil on medium or high heat. Remove meat and add the portabella mushrooms for five to seven minutes until somewhat reduced in size. Add the crushed tomatoes and the tomato paste. Stir until thoroughly combined. Season the mushroom tomato mixture to taste with sea salt and pepper, basil, oregano, balsamic vinegar and red wine. Put the hardest vegetables on the bottom of a large deep pot (carrots, new potatoes). Pour the can of beef broth and slurry* over the top (no water if cooking in crock pot). Now add the tomato mushroom mixture and then the beef. Finally add the button mushrooms (Kristin likes fresh spinach on top). Put lid on top. Do not stir. Let this cook for at least two hours on low heat. With a long wooden spoon, gently combine the stew, being careful not to break the vegetables. Continue cooking until a fork is easily inserted into a large potato. Eat.

*Slurry – ½ cup of water to 1 T of corn starch. Mix up with a fork so that there are no lumps.

OTHER

BASIC SALAD DRESSING

- 1 t salt
- ¼ t black pepper
- 1 t dry mustard
- Dash of Tabasco (optional)
- ¼ cup lemon juice
- 2/3 cup olive oil

Mix well and store in the refrigerator.

CAESAR SALAD DRESSING

Dr. Monk

- 1 cup organic mayonnaise
- 1 large fresh whole egg
- 1/2 cup shredded parmesan cheese
- 2 t extra virgin olive oil
- 2 T lemon juice
- 2 T anchovy paste (optional)
- 3 cloves of fresh garlic pressed (adjust to taste)
- 1/2 t fresh ground pepper
- 1/2 t dried parsley flakes
- 2 T horseradish

In a food processor or mixing bowl combine all ingredients except the olive oil. Combine to a creamy consistency and slowly pour the oil to thicken. Makes approximately two cups.

MAYONNAISE

- 1 egg
- 2 T lemon juice
- 1 cup olive oil

- 1 t mustard
- ¼ t powdered kelp (optional)
- ¼ t sea salt
- Seasonings (any herbs or spices you like)

Beat egg in blender on low speed. While continuing to blend slowly, add lemon juice and seasonings (optional), and then slowly drizzle in oil. Blend until the mixture is smooth. Because this mayonnaise has no vinegar, it will only store for a few days in the refrigerator so use it soon.

With mayonnaise you are now able to make salads like tuna, ham, or egg. Add these to greens for a healthy, low-carbohydrate lunch.

.

TRACKING SHEETS

WEIGHT LOSS SUMMARY: Weight loss goes way beyond counting calories. To insure that weight loss is both effective and healthy, one must correct the **BIG 3: hormonal imbalances, inflammation, and toxic tissues.** This means using a combination of diet, nutritional supplementation, and proper low-heart-rate exercise. Other helpful factors include tracking your progress and group participation for accountability and motivation.

TREATMENT SUMMARY: Losing weight is a process that will positively affect all aspects of your being. However, the ride can sometimes be a bit bumpy. Our treatments are designed to reduce stress at every level (structural, chemical and emotional) thereby making the journey much smoother. It is recommended that regular visits be scheduled in advance over the course of 3 or more months.

DIET SUMMARY: Simply put, the best diet is one that builds the immune system. Building the immune system takes care of the **BIG 3**. Diets that rely on low-calorie processed foods will not build the immune system and therefore will have a detrimental effect in the long run. Avoid sabotaging your immune system with food.

SUPPLEMENTATION SUMMARY: It will be necessary to incorporate quality supplements into your weight loss routine. This will replenish nutritional reserves, correct deficiencies and insure that adequate amounts of nutrients are present for the necessary metabolic changes. A sample schedule for MediClear is provided.

EXERCISE SUMMARY: Build your aerobic base by strictly exercising for 3 months within your target heart rate range. Exercise will most likely consist of walking 5 or more times per week for 40 or more minutes. Be sure to include a warm up, stretching and cool down period. Also, be sure to perform a maximum aerobic function (MAF) test at least every 4 weeks.

TOXICITY SELF TEST

POINT SCALE:
0 = NEVER OR ALMOST NEVER have the symptom
1 = OCCASIONALLY have it, effect is NOT SEVERE
2 = OCCASIONALLY have it, effect is SEVERE
3 = FREQUENTLY have it, effect is NOT SEVERE
4 = FREQUENTLY have it, effect is SEVERE

Rate each of the following symptoms based upon your health profile for the past 30 days

NOSE	SKIN
____ Stuffy nose	____ Acne
____ Sinus problems	____ Hives, rashes, dry skin
____ Hay fever	____ Hair loss
____ Sneezing attacks	____ Flushing or hot flashes
____ Excessive mucus	____ Excessive sweating
____ *TOTAL*	____ *TOTAL*
DIGESTIVE SYSTEM	**WEIGHT**
____ Nausea or vomiting	____ Binge eating / drinking
____ Diarrhea	____ Craving certain foods
____ Constipation	____ Excessive weight
____ Belching, passing gas	____ Compulsive eating
____ Bloated feeling	____ Water retention
____ Heartburn	____ Underweight
____ *TOTAL*	____ *TOTAL*
LUNGS	**EMOTIONS**
____ Chest congestion	____ Mood swings
____ Asthma, bronchitis	____ Anxiety, fear, nervous
____ Shortness of breath	____ Anger, irritability
____ Difficulty breathing	____ Depression
____ *TOTAL*	____ *TOTAL*

EARS	JOINTS / MUSCLES
____ Itchy ears	____ Pain or aches in joints
____ Ear aches, ear infection	____ Arthritis
____ Drainage from ear	____ Stiffness
____ Ringing in ears	____ Pain or aches in muscles
____ Hearing loss	____ Weakness / Tiredness
____ *TOTAL*	____ *TOTAL*
HEART	**OTHER**
____ Skipped heartbeats	____ Frequent illness
____ Chest pain	____ Frequent or urgent urination
____ Rapid heartbeats	____ Genital itch, discharge
____ *TOTAL*	____ *TOTAL*
MIND	**MOUTH / THROAT**
____ Poor memory	____ Chronic coughing
____ Confusion	____ Frequent gagging
____ Poor concentration	____ Need to clear throat
____ Poor coordination	____ Sore throat, hoarse
____ Difficulty making decisions	____ Swollen or discolored tongue, gums, lips
____ Stuttering, stammering	____ Canker sores
____ Slurred speech	____ *TOTAL*
____ Learning disabilities	
____ *TOTAL*	

Figure XVII

Score	Level of Toxicity
<20	Not significant
20-50 or 10+ in any one section	Mild
50-100	Moderate
100+	Severe

MEDICLEAR

This is a powerful supplement that will change your body for the better. There is the chance that MediClear may work too quickly. Therefore, we suggest gradually increasing the dosage and then leveling off (see: example below)

If you scored higher than 50 on the Toxicity Questionnaire begin with 1/3 or 1/2 scoop and work your way up.

Here is an example of how to get started:

	Breakfast	Lunch	Dinner
Build up	1 scoop		
Build up	1 scoop	1 scoop	
Build up	1 scoop	1 scoop	1 scoop
Build up	2 scoops	1 scoop	1 scoop
Build up	2 scoops	2 scoops	1 scoop
	Some may be able to complete the build up stage in less than one week. Many, however, may take much longer. Continue building up as long as it takes.		
Peak Stage	2 scoops	2 scoops	2 scoops
	Stay at peak stage for at least 3 days then begin staging down.		
Stage down	1 scoop	2 scoops	2 scoops
Stage down	1 scoop	1 scoop	2 scoops
Maintenance	1 scoop	1 scoop	1 scoop
	Maintenance can last for up to 6 months.		

Figure XVIII

TARGET HEART RATE

180- ______ +/- ______ = ______
AGE (SEE BELOW)

- Recovering from a major illness, surgery or taking daily medication.....**subtract 10**
- Have not exercised before, or have exercised but have been injured or are regressing, or experience frequent colds, flu, or under high stress.....**subtract 5**
- Exercising for up to two years without any real problems, and have not had colds or flu more than once or twice per year.....**subtract 0**
- Exercising for more than two years without any real problems and have been making progress in your program or competition.....**add 5**

Use your calculated target heart rate number as the high end of your heart rate range. Example: if your number is 138 bpm, then your fat burning heart rate range is 128 bpm -138 bpm.

MAXIMUM AEROBIC FUNCTION TEST

WHILE TRAINING IN YOUR HEART RATE RANGE:

- Pick an amount of time you are going to exercise and measure how far you go. Or,
- Pick a measured distance and record your time.
- If you are not improving, evaluate your health. Have you been:
    - Sick?
    - Stressed?
    - Getting Enough Rest?
    - Eating Bad Foods?

DATE	TIME	DISTANCE
01/01/03	**40**	**?**
01/31/03	**40**	**?**

DATE	TIME	DISTANCE
01/01/03	**?**	**3 MILES**
01/31/03	**?**	**3 MILES**

Perform a MAF test every 3 or 4 weeks.

PROGRESS TRACKING SHEET

DATE	WEIGHT	BMI	HIP/WAIST

Check each of the above every 4 weeks.

BMI

(WEIGHT ÷ HEIGHT (IN)^2) X 704.5

A BMI of 30 or more is considered obese and
a BMI between 25 to 29.9 is considered overweight.

HIP TO WAIST RATIO

Waist measurement ÷ Hip measurement

Women with waist-to-hip ratios of more than 0.8 are at increased health risk because of their fat distribution

Men with waist-to-hip ratios of more than 1.0 are at increased health risk because of their fat distribution

TESTIMONIALS

Below are testimonials from just a few of the chronically ill people I have been able to help with the techniques discussed in this book. I hope you find their stories inspiring.

Hi Dr. Monk. I just wanted to tell you how great I feel since I went to you. I had suffered for years with allergies and sinus problems, with no real relief. I am 31 now, and I can remember going to the doctor with sinus infections, allergies, and upper respiratory problems since I was 7 or 8 years old. All the MD's did for me was to prescribe antihistimines for the allergies, decongestants for the sinuses, and antibiotics if I had an infection. I was basically healthy years ago, as I was on the wrestling team in school, and later competed in powerlifting and bodybuilding. I watched my diet very closely and my problems were not constant and were pretty much bearable until a couple of years ago, when I had gotten really slack in my workouts and diet. I was working long hours (12 hour shifts, sometimes 60 or more hours per week), and eating junk food and drinking soft drinks all the time. I started feeling really run down and had more severe sinus and allergy problems. It got to the point where every time it rained or the temperature changed, I was having migraines and very serious sinus headaches and congestion. My sinuses were chronically congested and I was getting extremely cold natured, to the point where I could not stand to be around air conditioning. I was having about 3-4 migraine headaches per week. Also, I was having abdominal cramps, indigestion, and general digestive discomfort on a regular basis. I started working out again, but found that I was not recovering from my workouts like I used to and minor injuries were really slow to heal. I was PRAYING for a cure. Then, I found a section in an old book about candida and leaky gut syndrome. I read it and started thinking that candida could be what was causing my problems. Then, I had a really terrible migraine one day, and I decided that I had enough. I got on the internet and started researching candida heavily, and noticed that all of my symptoms were candida / leaky gut related. I found a link to your website on a personal testimonial site about candida recovery. After my first visit with you, and starting the supplement and diet plan to eliminate candida, I felt pretty bad for about 2 days (detox symptoms from candida die-off), then I noticed something. I started to feel much better. MY HEAD DIDN'T HURT AND MY NOSE WASN'T STUFFED UP for the first time in YEARS. I did not deviate from the diet at all except for about 3 weeks into it I had about a half teaspoon of hot sauce while eating out. I also didn't miss a single dose of the supplements. So, basically I have been free from migraine headaches, sinus, and allergy problems ever since my second day on the program. IT REALLY WORKS. If someone is reading this and is skeptical, I would say to them that going to Dr. Monk was best thing I ever did for my health. It has been about eight weeks now, and I feel totally fantastic and am 100% free of symptoms.

Thank you for all your help!

D. Williams

Dear Scott,

For over three years I had been having sharp shooting pains in my left kidney area. I tried a variety of treatments to no avail. After an automobile accident in January I made an appointment to see Dr. Scott Monk based on a friend's referral.

Dr. Monk tested the kidney and confirmed that it was in crisis and suggested a supplement to cleanse and support the kidneys. Within a few weeks the pain in my kidney was completely gone.

I shutter to think what could have happened if it weren't for the treatment I received from Dr. Monk. His ability to interpret the body's signals that something is wrong and respond appropriately to heal the source of the pain and not just mask it are rare gifts.

I would highly recommend Dr. Monk for whatever ails you.

Cathy Fuss

I could tell quite a story about my health and how I have benefited from Dr. Monk's services in the last three weeks, but I'd rather keep this short. I've gained twenty-five pounds in the last two years. At age thirty-nine the thought of gaining any more concerned me. Dealing with depression, sinus congestion, achy joints and mood swings over the last ten to twelve years has caused me to search within and beyond traditional medicine support for answers. I've tried to guess if "foods" that I ate might be the culprit of my concerns. That's been an overwhelming task to decipher on my own.

Through AK Dr. Monk identified a **severe wheat allergy** and choose to focus on other areas of nutritional health as well. I'll let him explain. Within a week I had more energy and felt like exercising. I was able to seek out organic foods and begin to eat whole foods. Two weeks into this I felt better than I had in twenty years. Then came a holiday, baking cookies for my kids and oops, I ate a cookie. Yes it had wheat. It lead to not feeling great and craving cookies and chips. The following visit to Dr. Monk found me yawning, dragging, listless and tired. The cookie was a test. Now I definitely have answers.

All those years I thought food might be the root of some physical problems. It's true. It was. Food was a culprit in my dwindling health. Following Dr. Monk's personalized plan for me has resulted in the **elimination of**, achy joints, hemorrhoids, mild incontinence, sleepless restless nights, PMS, disorganized thinking, cravings for chocolate and junk food, achy sinus congestion, and weight gain. My husband has commented, "I like the new you." My daughters have commented that I'm much more calm and focused. Life is coming into balance at this time through intestinal cleansing, reducing stress, refocusing on my spiritual growth as a Christian, and eating whole foods that were designed to be of nutritional value to me. I never separate God's presence from my health or vise versa. This has been a really healthy time for me physically and spiritually. Eating in a new way will be a lifelong journey. Thank you, Dr. Monk for your dedication to this profession. This is truly a blessing in my life.

Jane W.

ADDITIONAL SOURCES

BUSINESSES

Nationally

Grain Mills	Health for You. PO Box 180327 Utica, MI 48318-0327 (810) 798-0849 1-877-MOM-BAKE FAX: (810) 798-0839
Kefir Grains	G.E.M. Cultures (707) 964-2922
Piima	Send your mailing information along with a $5 check for one packet or a $20 check for five packets to: Piima, PO Box 2614, La Mesa, CA 91943
Sea Salt	Grain and Salt Society. (800) 867-7258
Wheat	Wheat Montana. (800)-535-2798

WEBSITES

General Health

http://candidarecovery.terrashare.com	Karen Trip's website discussing her struggles with Candidiasis and how she was healed. Great information and recipes.
www.alternativemedicine.com	This is a great site for alternative health information and resources.
www.chetday.com	Chet Day's website discussing how he overcame cancer through nutrition, exercise and many other treatments.
www.drdavidwilliams.com	Dr. Williams travels the globe in search of highly effective herbal cures and treatments that have been used in remote parts of the world for centuries.
www.drweil.com	Dr. Andrew Weil, an M.D., has become well known as an advocate for alternative medicine.
www.drwhitaker.com	Dr. Whitaker, a well known M.D. uses many alternative approaches in his practice and is the author of, <u>A Guide To Natural Healing</u>.
www.healthy.net	Health World Online. This is a great place to look for information about specific conditions. There is a great deal of helpful information.
www.johnleemd.com	Dr. John Lee's website. Go here for information regarding

	hormone replacement therapy, osteoporosis and breast cancer.
www.mercola.com	Dr. Joseph Mercola's website. Go here for information regarding vaccines.
www.choosehealth.net	My website. Contact me for an appointment, take our online health test or simply learn more about the topics in this book.
www.saveyourlifevideos.com	Cancer curing videos by an unorthodox doctor (my favorite kind).
www.teachhealth.com	A great site that explains stress in an easy to understand way. Complete with a stress evaluation and enjoyable illustrations.
www.thyroid.about.com	Mary Shomon's Thyroid Guide. Everything you want to know about the thyroid gland.

Health Research

http:jama.ama-assn.org	Journal of the American Medical Association
www.bmj.com	British Medical Journal
www.cdc.gov	Center for Disease Control
www.health.harvard.edu	Harvard Health
www.medline.com	Medline
www.nejm.org	New England Journal of Medicine
www.thelancet.com	The Lancet

Food/Cooking

www.homehealthresource.net	a.k.a. Herb Plenty. Go here to purchase juicers and grain mills. They also have great links to all

	things pioneer like.
www.healthforyouministry.com/	The place to go to find grain mills, bread machines and other at home necessities.
www.sweetvia.com	A very sweet site. Learn all about stevia, one of the sweetest herbs around.
www.westonaprice.org/	A site devoted to the work of Dr. Weston A. Price, whose ideas about health and nutrition are a180 degrees departure from today's pseudoscience.
www.wheatmontana.com	A good resource to learn about and purchase grains of all kinds.

Miscellaneous

www.el.com	Essential Links. Hundreds of links to almost anything you want to find.
www.naturallyhealthy.org	Shonda Parker's website. A great place for mothers and those who are expecting.
www.christianbest.com	Over 2000 links to anything Christian.

BOOKS

Chronic Illness

Definitive Guide to Cancer
W. John Diamond
W. Lee Cowden
Burton Goldberg

A must read for any person suffering from cancer who would like to know about alternative therapies or ways of boosting their immune system. After reading this book you will gain a whole new perspective on some of the abuses in our medical system.

The Complete Book of Essential Oils and Aromatherapy
Valerie Ann Worwood

Essential oils can heal cuts, remove emotional stress, and even make the house smell pretty. Learn to use these oils in place of other household items.

Winning the War Against Asthma and Allergies
Ellen Cutler

Learn about an effective way to completely eliminate allergies and asthma for a lifetime…N.A.E.T. I use a version of this protocol in my office to help patients with lifelong problems.

Your Bodies Many Cries For Water
F. Batmanghelidj

Sometimes what we need the most has always been within reach.

Diet/Cooking

Cook Right For Your Type Dr. Peter J. D'Adamo	Many good recipes and guidelines. Certain foods are selected according to blood type.
Nourishing Traditions Sally Fallon	This is quickly becoming one of my favorite books. I make reference to it in the Maintenance & Prevention chapter. This should be in everyone's kitchen!
The Body Ecology Diet Donna Gates	The best book by far for coping with yeast related problems and for building better health through diet.
The Miracle of Fasting Paul C. Bragg	Learn about the benefits of fasting. I do not agree with the author's theology but his fasting principles are excellent.

Fitness/Exercise

In Fitness and In Health Phil Maffetone	The name says it all. This book covers all the basics and enough detail to make the reader well informed.
The Maffetone Method Phil Maffetone	The holistic, low-stress, no-pain way to exceptional fitness. Dr. Maffetone's latest book. All the best of his other exercise and fitness books plus a great deal more. Great for long time and beginning exercisers.

Motherhood

Mommy Diagnostics Shonda Parker	A great book to help mom with common aliments. Many practical tips.
The Naturally Healthy Pregnancy Shonda Parker	A terrific book to help mothers understand the gift and responsibility of pregnancy. Written by a first child, C-section mother who went on to deliver the rest of her children naturally.

Parenthood / Kids Health

Beyond Antibiotics Michael Schmidt	A good book for parents or anyone who is concerned about the negative effects of antibiotics. It provides a clear understanding of the short and long-term effects of one of the most prescribed medicines today.
Pregnancy to Parenthood Linda Goldberg	A resource guide to help parents with questions before and during child rearing.
Shepherding a Child's heart Tedd Tripp	Why do so many parents have out-of-control children? This book provides a Biblical response to today's poor attempts at child rearing.
The Infants Survival Guide Lendon H. Smith	An explanation for S.I.D.S.? What about vaccines, antibiotics, etc? This is A MUST READ for all, not just parents!
The Vaccine Guide : Making an Informed Choice Randall Neustaedter	Vaccinations could be one of the most controversial topics in health today. Learn both sides

before making your decision.

To Train up a Child
Michael and Debbie Pearl

Another spectacular book. This book definitely runs counter-culture to what we are bombarded with today regarding the raising of children. However, once read, a parent will begin to understand the true nature inside the heart of every child and how to properly guide them.

Reference

Prescription for Nutritional Healing
James F. Blach M.D.
Phyllis A. Blach C.N.C

Practical A-Z reference to drug-free remedies Using Vitamins, minerals, herbs & food supplements. The well-known resource for natural treatments of a vast array of conditions. It should be a part of the library of every home.

Encyclopedia of Nutritional Medicine
Murray / Pizzorno

A complete reference book detailing many conditions with their nutritional corrections.

Spiritual

Fasting for the Spiritual Breakthrough
Elmer L. Towns

Understand the process and importance of fasting, not just for physical, but spiritual well being.

The Case For Christ
Lee Strobel

Is there actual evidence that we can examine to determine if Jesus is who he said he was? Or are millions of Christians simply ignorant and unscientific? The answer to these questions will change your life forever.

The Case For Faith
Lee Strobel

Lee Strobel examines the hard questions that make God look very unimpressive. Why is there so much suffering in the world? How can a loving God send people to hell forever?

The Face That Demonstrates The Farce of Evolution
Hank Hanegraaff

No other theory or idea has done so much harm. Evolution is responsible for more than 120 million deaths in the 20th century alone! Find out why this theory is nothing more than bad science.

The Power of a Praying Parent
Stormie Omartian

Proper parenting is the toughest job in the universe. This book helps the helpless parent by encouraging them through the power of godly prayer.

Women's Health

What Your Doctor May Not Tell You About Menopause
Dr. John Lee

The breakthrough book on natural progesterone. Hormone replacement therapy is rampant in our country for women over fifty. This book reveals many frightening facts about the dangers of HRT.

What Your Doctor May Not Tell You About Premenopause
Dr. John Lee

Balance your hormones and your life from 30 to 50. Dr. Lee's follow-up book helps younger women avoid hormonal problem starting now.

BIBLIOGRAPHY

Atkins, Robert C., M.D. *Dr Atkins' New Diet Revolution.* New York: Avon Books, 1992.

Balch, James, M.D., Balch, Phyllis A. C.N.C. *Prescription for Nutritional Healing.* Avery Publishing Group, Inc., 1990.

Bates, Donna. *The Body Ecology Diet.*

Batmanghelidj, F. *Your Bodies many Cries For Water.* Global Health Solutions Inc. 1997.

Behe, Michael J. *Darwin's Black Box.* New York: The Free Press, 1996.

Biser, Sam. *Curing With Cayenne and its Herbal Partners.* Save Your Life Videos, 1999.

Block, Mary Ann. *No More Ritalin.* Kensington Health, 1996.

Boyll, Dale. *Good Health God's Way.* Scriputal Nutrition Press. Spring Hill: 1999.

Chapman-Smith, David. *The Chiropractic Profession.* NCMIC Group, 2000.

Colgan, Michael. *Optimum Sports Nutrition.* Advanced Research Press, 1993.

Connolly, Pat. *The Candida Albicans Yeast-Free Cookbook.*

Cutler, Ellen. *Winning the War Against Allergies and Asthma.* Delmar Publishers, 1998.

D'Adamo, Peter J. *Cook Right for Your Blood Type.* Putnum Publishing, 1998.

Diamond, John, M.D., Cowden, Lee, M.D., Goldberg, Burton. *An Alternative Medicine Definitive Guide to Cancer.* Future Medicine Publishing, 1997.

Durlacher, James, D.C. *Freedom From Fear Forever.* Van Ness Publishing. Mesa: 2000.

Fallon, Sally. *Nourishing Traditions.* New Trends Publishing, 1999

Gerber, Richard, M.D.. *Vibrational Medicine.* Bear and Company. Santa Fe: 1996.

Gordon, Deborah, M.D., Siple, Molly. *Menopause, The Natural Way.* John Wiley and Sons Inc.:2001.

Harley, Susan. *Gentle Hands.* Awesome Books Publishing, 2000.

Hawkins, David R., M.D. *Power vs. Force.* Hay House, Inc., 2002.

Lee, John, M.D. *What Your Doctor May Not Tell You About Menopause.* Warner Books, 1996.

Lipski, Elizabeth. *Digestive Wellness.* Keats Publishing, 1996.

Lundberg, George, M.D. *Severed Trust, Why American Medicine Hasn't Been Fixed.* Basic Books, 2000.

Maffetone, Philip, D.C. *In Fitness and in Health.* David Barmore Productions, 2002.

Maffetone, Philip, D.C. *Training for Endurance.* David Barmore Productions, 1996.

Meyerowitz, Steven. *Juice Fasting and Detoxification.* The Sprout House, 1996

Mondoa, Emil, M.D. *Sugars That Heal.* Ballantine Books, New York: 2001.

Mueller, Rudolph, M.D. *As Sick As It Gets.* Olin Fredrick Inc. New York: 2001.

Neustaedter, Randall. *The Vaccine Guide : Making an Informed Choice.*

Parker, Shonda. *Mommy Diagnostics.* Loyal Publishing, 1998

Parker, Shonda. *The Naturally Healthy Pregnancy.* Loyal Publishing, 1996.

Pearl, Michael. *To Train up a Child.* Michael and Debbie Pearl, 1999.

Pelton, Ross, RPh, PhD, CCN. *Drug-Induced Nutrient Depletion Handbook.* Lexi-Comp, Inc. NHR, 2000.

Rogers, Sherry, M.D. *The Scientific Basis for Selected Environmental Techniques.* SK Publishing, 1994.

Rogers, Sherry, M.D. *Tired or Toxic.* Prestige Publishing, 1990.

Rondberg, Terry A., D.C. *Chiropractic First.* The Chiropractic

Journal, 1996.

Sahley, Billie Jay. *Control Hyperactivity A.D.D. Naturally.* Pain & Stress Publications, 1997.

Schmidt, Michael; Smith, Lendon; Sehnert, Keith. *Beyond Antibiotics*, North Atlantic Books, 1994.

Schmitt, Walter, D.C.. *Complied Notes on Clinical Nutrition.* David Barmore Productions, 1990.

Sears, Barry, Ph.D. *Mastering The Zone.* ReganBooks, 1997.

Sears, Barry, Ph.D. *The Age Free Zone.* ReganBooks, 1999.

Smith, Lendon H. *The Infants Survival Guide.*

Tourles, Stephanie. *The Herbal Body Book.* Storey Publishing, 1994.

Towns, Elmer. *Fasting For A Spiritual Breakthrough.* Regal Books, 1996.

Walther, David S. *Applied Kinesiology, Synopsis 2nd Ed.* Systems DC, 2000.

Wiley, T.S.; Formby, Bent. *Lights Out.* Pocket Books, 2000.

INDEX

A

Adrenal Glands.. 14, 33, 38, 57, 58, 59 - 63, 78, 79, 80, 91, 92, 95, 152, 155, 177, 188, 199, 219
Adrenal Stress Index57, 60, 80
Aerobic Exercise 38, 219, 225
Aerobic System 38, 217, 218
Allergic Reaction 73
Correction Of 180
Allergies..... 17, 151, 273
Alternative Health Philosophy 2
Anti Oxidants.......... 160
Antibiotics 115, 236
Antibodies 69, 191, 207, 208
Applied Kinesiology 23
Arteriosclerosis ... 9, 198
Asthma....................... 24

B

Beliefs
Alternative Health Care . 3
Traditional Health Care..3
Birth Control Pills85, 86
The Effects Of................. 86
Birth Defects 188, 189
Body Mass Index (BMI) 129, 130, 264
Body
Listening To.................. 148
Body Fluid 213
Body Mass Index..... 129
Breakfast................... 261
Breast Milk....... 191, 192
Breast Milk.............. 192

C

Candida ... 44, 66, 72, 91, 103, 114, 115, 116, 160, 199, 235, 236, 278
Correction..................... 117
Die Off........................... 116
Candidiasis 270
Carbohydrate Intolerance (CI)... 104
Carbohydrates 104, 105, 141, 142, 195
Carotenoids 196
Catabolism............... 133
Catecholamines 80

Causes Of Hormonal Imbalances 90
Cayenne Pepper...... 161
Cell................. 9, 14, 163
Celtic Sea Salt.......... 152
Chemicals 236
Cholesterol 72, 107, 109, 143, 154, 199
Cholesterol Correction 109
Cholic Acid............. 107
Chronic Fatigue 114, 228
Chronic Illness Protocol 65
Carbohydrate Intolerance (CI) . 104, 105, 106
Colic......................... 203
Colon Cleansing 162
Colonics 163
Common Cold......... 215
Cool Down 223, 258
Corpus Luteum......... 89
Cortisol................ 59, 79
Cough Syrup 186
Cranial Bones 34, 36, 37, 203
Cranial Faults........... 36
Cross-Crawl.............. 29

D

Dehydration 9
Depression.... 21, 92, 96, 105, 131, 132, 182, 259
Depression Symptoms 96
Desensitization... 66, 72, 75, 117
Detoxification 44, 47, 48, 157, 158, 159, 170, 187
At Home 157
Supplements For.......... 160
DHEA 59
Diet
Yeast 234
Digestive Support ... 184
Disc Injuries............. 122
Disease Model 1, 8
Dural Tension........... 34
Dysbiosis.................... 68

E

Ear Infections........... 204
Eggs . 111, 193, 195, 197, 237
Electromagnetic Fields 53
EMF's 53
Enemas 162
Enzymes 160
Epinephrine 80
Equal®..................... 235
Essential Fatty Acids 160
Estrogen .. 58, 70, 84, 85, 86, 87, 88, 89, 90, 91, 93, 95, 100, 102, 103, 106, 107, 115, 136, 194
Estrogen Balance..... 102
Estrogen Dominance 93
Eustachian Tube...... 205
Exercise 49, 159, 161, 216, 219, 274
Ezekiel Bread........... 197

F

Fallon, Sally 193
Fasting...................... 169

Fat...... 38, 110, 216, 217, 218, 219, 220
Fat-Free Foods 110
Partially Hydrogenated 154
Saturated 110, 143, 196
Trans-Fats 160
Fats
Chart 146
Saturated 143
FATS......................... 143
Hydrogenated.............. 144
Fatty Acids...... 166, 192, 195, 223
Female Sexual Cycle. 87
Fever......................... 215
Fiber.......................... 142
Fibromyalgia .. 136, 158, 228
Fight Or Flight Reaction................. 78
Filtered Water 152, 162, 171
Fitness 216, 217
Flax Oil...................... 166
Flax Seed Oil............ 172
Follicle Stimulating Hormone 89
Follicle Stimulating Hormone (FSH)... 87, 89
Food
Preparation Of 171
Food Allergens 138, 174
Food Allergies 9, 32, 66, 68, 70, 86, 98, 116, 137, 138, 180, 204, 205
Food Reactions........ 211
Formulas.................. 193
Free Radicals 160
Fruit.......... 197, 199, 202
Functional Illness.1, 12, 22, 57
Fungal Infections 91, 215

G

Gallbladder Flush ... 166
Gastro-Intestinal Tract 67
General Adaptive Syndrome 58
Glucocorticoids ... 58, 79
Golgi Tendon Organs 26
Gonadotropin-Releasing Hormone (Gnrh) 87
Grain Mills 172
Grains 152, 155, 171, 173, 193, 196, 197, 272
Soaking.......................... 172
Grains .. 70, 83, 103, 104, 112, 171, 172
Grated Liver 194
Gut Permeability 74

H

Heart Disease ... 6, 8, 20, 110, 160
Heart Rate Monitor 221, 225
Heavy Metal Poisoning 66
High Blood Pressure.. 8, 9, 169
High Protein Diet...... 44
High-Fructose Foods 200
Hip To Waist Ratio . 264
Hormone Replacement Therapy (HRT) 84

Hormones 62, 79, 85, 131, 152
DHEA 59
Cortisol 59, 79
Epinephrine 80
Estrogen .. 58, 70, 84, 85, 86, 87, 88, 89, 90, 91, 93, 95, 100, 102, 103, 106, 107, 115, 136, 194
Gonadotropin-Releasing Hormone (Gnrh) 87
Glucocorticoids ... 58, 79
Luteinizing Hormone (LH) 87
Progesterone .. 88, 90, 277
Serotonin. 96, 97, 98, 105, 182
Sex Hormones 58
Follicle Stimulating Hormone (FSH) ... 87, 89
Hot Flashes 95, 131
HRT 84, 85, 86, 91
Human Body 9
Hyperinsulinemia ... 131
Hypoglycemia Correction 106
Hypothyroidism 60

I

Iatrogenic 6
Ige 73
Igg 73
Immune Response 75
Immune System. 13, 38, 48, 58, 110, 144, 158, 162, 187, 191, 200, 213, 219, 273
Immune System. 12, 45, 53, 54, 66, 67, 68, 73, 74, 75, 76, 79, 115, 116, 137, 138, 175, 178, 188, 208, 209, 212, 214, 215, 226, 257
Immune System
The Breaking Of 154
The Building Of 151
Infection .. 66, 67, 69, 97, 114, 115, 116, 164, 178, 205, 208, 212, 214, 215, 236, 260
Inflammation ... 133, 179
Correction Of 179
Injury Recall Technique (IRT) 27
Innate Intelligence 10
Insulin Resistance .. 106, 132, 141
Insulin Resistance Syndrome 131
International College Of Applied Kinesiology 23
Irritable Bowel Formula 165
Isoflavones 102

J

Juices 200

K

Kefir. 193, 196, 197, 201, 202, 235
Kidney
Cleansing 168

L

Lactose 142
Leaky Gut Syndrome68

L-Glutamine ... 161, 162, 166, 213
Ligans ... 103
Liver
Cleansing ... 166
Disease ... 199
Low Back Pain ... 121
Low Back Pain
Causes Of ... 123
Correction Of ... 124
Low Blood Sugar ... 104
Luteinizing Hormone (LH) ... 87

M

Macronutrients 43, 104, 140, 141, 148, 160
Macronutrients . 43, 140
MAF Test ... 224
Manual Muscle Testing ... 23
Margarine ... 111
Maximum Aerobic Function Test (MAF) ... 224
Meat Stocks ... 152
Medications (Anti-Depressives) ... 98
Mediclear ... 261
Menopause .. 92, 95, 279
Menstrual Cycle. 18, 21, 87, 95, 115
Menstrual Irregularities ... 93
Microorganisms 67, 103
Migraine Headaches 36, 227
Milk . 101, 152, 154, 174, 183, 185, 194
Mineralcorticoids ... 58
Minerals ... 43, 45, 135, 140, 141, 154, 175, 177, 189, 192, 193, 198
Moodiness
Correction Of ... 182
MSG ... 155
Muscle Fibers ... 38, 218

N

Nambudripad Allergy Elimination Technique (N.A.E.T) ... 76
National Institutes Of Health (NIH) ... 84
Nervous System ... 10
Nervousness ... 9
Neural Tube Defect 188
Neuro Emotional Therapy (N.E.T.) ... 50
Neuro-Emotional Complex (N.E.C.) 50, 51
Neuro-Immune Treatment (NIT) . 226
Neurolymphatic Reflex ... 27
Neurolymphatic Reflexes ... 28
Neurovascular Reflex ... 27
Nutrasweet® ... 235
Nutritional Imbalances ... 9

O

Oatmeal ... 197
Obesity ... 28
Oligosaccharides ... 141
Organic Foods ... 187
Orthotics ... 40, 41
Osteoporosis ... 60, 218, 270

Osteoporosis............ 100
Over-Training ... 38, 219
Ovulation............. 88, 89

P

Pain.............. 19, 20, 118
Parathyroid.............. 101
Pesticides 192
Phytates........... 154, 172
Phytoestrogens........ 102
PMS 84, 92, 93
Pre Menstrual
Syndrome (PMS).. 93
Pressure Receptors ... 25
Probiotics 160, 162, 212, 213
Processed Foods 155, 192
Progesterone 88, 90, 277
Prostaglandins 143
Proteins 147
Digestion Of................ 148
Psyllium Husk 161, 162

Q

Qlink.............. 54, 55, 56

R

Recipes 237
Reciprocal Inhibition 26
Recovery Symptoms 71
Resistance 13, 14, 16, 218, 223

S

Sample Menu 201
Serotonin...... 96, 97, 98, 105, 182
Sex Hormones 58
Skin Cleansing 168
Skull...................... 34, 36
Sleep Cycles.............. 58
Snacking.................. 199
Sodas...........81, 101, 198
Sore Throat 215
Soups 196, 197, 237
Soy 110, 143, 154, 194
Soybeans 154
Spinal Adjustment.... 32
Spinal Misalignment 40
Spindle Cells............. 26
Sprouting 171
Stews........................ 197
Stimuli 11, 24, 26, 28
Stress 7, 9, 11, 13, 14, 16, 17, 20, 21, 29, 32, 33, 38, 48, 57, 58, 59, 62, 63, 67, 72, 77, 78, 100, 123, 148, 159, 192, 198, 216, 218, 219, 221, 223, 273, 274
Stress List 80
Stress Management... 80
Stress Priority 15
Stress Relief Tea 186
Stretching......... 223, 258
Subclinical Infection .65
Subluxation... 28, 32, 33, 34, 123
Sugar.... 58, 60, 110, 141, 152, 154, 198 - 200, 201, 202, 217, 220, 222, 236
Sunlight.................... 101
Supplements3, 9, 45, 46, 62, 63, 100, 116, 119, 126, 136, 138, 158, 160, 162, 164, 166, 167, 175, 190, 192, 212, 213, 226, 257, 276
Synthetic Fats 110

T

Target Heart Rate .. 220, 262
Teas 185
Thyroid ... 100, 102, 231, 271
Toxic Air 135
Toxic Food 135
Toxic Water 135
Toxicity 9, 11, 15, 18, 32, 42, 48, 72, 77, 134, 136, 158, 261
Symptoms Of 136
Toxicity Self Test..... 259
Toxins.. 9, 13, 47, 48, 60, 157, 158, 159, 160, 170, 192, 223
Traditional Medicine.. 5
Triglycerides... 105, 107, 108, 109, 111, 132, 143, 199
Tryptophan.... 96, 97, 98
Tyramine 98

V

Vaccinations 205
Vector Point Cranial Therapy 34
Vinegar 152, 235
Viscero-Somatic Reflexes 124
Vitamin B1 .... 45, 46
Vitamin C.. 26, 146, 200, 211
Vitamin C Powder . 200, 213
Vitamin Cofactors 97
Vitamins 45, 102, 166
Synthetic 155

W

Walking .. 9, 38, 219, 222
Warming Up 223
Weight Gain
Causes Of 127
Whole Milk Products 193

ORDER FORM

Infinity Publishing: Toll Free (877) BUY-BOOK
(610) 519-0261 Fax
www.buybooksontheweb.com

Dr. Monk: (303) 399-5117 Phone
(303) 399-5140 Fax
www.choosehealth.net
drmonk@choosehealth.net

Power Point presentations must be ordered directly from Dr. Monk. They are approximately 60 minutes in length and contain 75+ slides. They are heavily based on the book, Choose Health, which is the recommended resource.

	Qty.	Price	Total
Choose Health!		$18.95	
POWER POINT SLIDES			
Applied Kinesiology		$75.00	
Applied Kinesiology and Stress		$75.00	
Applied Kinesiology and Allergies		$75.00	
Caring for Children		$75.00	
Weight Loss Part I – The Metabolic Stumbling Blocks		$75.00	
Weight Loss Part II – Diet and Exercise		$75.00	
Women's Health		$75.00	
Any 3 Presentations		$175	
All 7 Presentations		$400	
Total			
Sales Tax 7.2% CO. residents only.			
$2.50 shipping for each book or any/all Power Point Presentation(s); $1.00 for each additional book.			
Grand Total			

NOTES

NOTES